# Everyday Techniques to Overcome Anxiety

## And Mental Health Struggles

Ira Bowman

FOREWORD BY Max Kayes

Janet Hogan, Dr. David Foster, Eric Rosen,
Jim Lomot, Lisa A. Jones, Rick Loek,
Ronita Godsi, Titia Niehorster,
Shmiko Cole, Tim Bowman

ISBN: 979-8-89079-053-8 (hardback)
ISBN: 979-8-89079-052-1 (paperback)
ISBN: 979-8-89079-054-5 (ebook)

# CONTENTS

# FOREWORD

BY
MAX KAYES

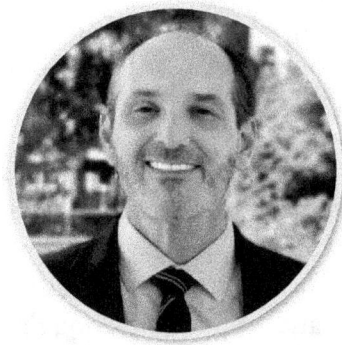

*"People grow five thousand roses in one garden, yet they don't find what they are looking for. And now, here is my secret. It's quite simple. One sees clearly only with the heart. Anything essential is invisible to the eyes."* (Saint-Exupery A. d., 1943)

*The Little Prince by Antoine de Saint- Exupéry*

Complexity often hinders our ability to execute effectively in various aspects of our lives. As the Little Prince astutely observed, humans are caught in a constant frenzy of haste and busyness, often lacking clarity about the outcomes they seek or their true purpose. With nearly 40 years of experience providing psychotherapy and coaching to individuals, couples, families, and business owners, I have discovered that unnecessary complexity often obscures the simplest solutions. The mind itself is primarily responsible for veiling these solutions. As our young friend wisely stated, "Anything essential is invisible to the eye."

The authors of *Everyday Techniques to Overcome Anxiety and Mental Health Strategies* aim to uncover simple, rather than complex, methods to reduce mental clutter and embrace the present moment, thus enhancing all aspects of our lives, relationships, and business endeavors. While the mind can be an incredible tool when used skillfully, its misuse can lead to disasters in business, relationships, and families. Why does this happen? It is because the mind seldom remains in the present moment.

The brain's primary function is not to bring us joy but to ensure our survival. Nonetheless, our brain possesses remarkable capabilities, regulating vital biological functions such as the heart, lungs, and hormone balance. Additionally, it governs our interpretation and response to thoughts.

However, when faced with a perceived threat, we instinctively enter the fight-flight-freeze response to protect ourselves. This state triggers the production of powerful hormones and chemicals in our body, preparing us for defense against any perceived danger, whether real or purely psychological.

Conversely, when we perceive safety or positivity, our body responds by producing chemicals and allowing the flow of neurotransmitters that promote feelings of well-being. Nonetheless, the body reacts to what the mind perceives as reality, blurring the line between thoughts and actual events. By referring to the mind, I am referring to the habitual patterns of thought we engage with automatically. These patterns occur unconsciously, and we are no longer in a conscious state momentarily.

It is estimated that we have anywhere between 6,200 (Poppenk, 2020) and 60,000 thoughts (National Science Foundation, 2005) or evaluations by the mind each day. Unfortunately, these thoughts are often the same ones from the previous day, which do not empower us but diminish our joy in living and our ability to live in the present moment.

Patterns of thoughts rooted in the past can evoke feelings of sadness, anger, resentment, and regret as they continuously resurface in the present moment. Similarly, focusing on the future often leads to mild anxiety or overwhelming uncertainty, triggering panic reactions or panic attacks. What people experience as life is more like the portrayal of a computer-generated existence in the movie The Matrix.

But what are you truly seeking? Most individuals yearn for peace, joy, and certainty, which are states that transcend thought. René Descartes, the renowned philosopher, scientist, and mathematician, famously wrote in 1637, "Cogito, ergo sum," or "I think; therefore, I am." However, a richer experience of life and understanding can be attained by consciously being without the constant chatter of thought. One can be conscious without thought.

Throughout this discussion, the authors will explore utilizing our senses, breathing, walking, and meditation as practices that do not rely on thought. If you anticipate finding complex strategies, you may be disappointed. Please remember while reading that the authors are industry leaders in applied sciences, academia, coaching, education, media, and philanthropy.

I am truly honored to have been asked to write the introduction to this book and humbled to stand beside their great accomplishments. They encourage you to embrace simplicity. The returns on investing in these simple practices are profound.

The term simple originated from its etymology, meaning plain, sweet, without duplicity, which is whole. (Harper, 2003) You receive a true gift by applying the straightforward suggestions the authors offer, who aim to assist you by sharing their journeys. They desire to serve you to go beyond the ordinary to find the extraordinary that is right under the surface, "invisible to the eye."

I often remind my clients that things are simple but not easy. Adopting new habits requires repetition and persistence. Therefore, be patient with yourself as you try these new strategies and resist the urge to be critical. Approach them with gentleness and self-compassion. Let these experts guide you. You are in good hands.

## References

Harper, D. (2003). *https://www.etymonline.com/word/Simple*. Retrieved from https://www.etymonline.com: https://www.etymonline.com/word/Simple

Hatfield, G. (2014). *Renee Descartes*. Retrieved from Stanford Encyclopedia of Philosophy: https://plato.stanford.edu/entries/descartes/#Bib

*National Science Foundation*. (2005). Retrieved from nsf.gov.

Poppenk, J. T. (2020). Brain meta-state transitions demarcate thoughts across task contexts exposing the mental noise of trait neuroticism. *Nature Communications*.

Saint-Exupery, A. d. (1943). *The Little Prince*. New York: Harper Collins.

# Walking It Off –
# More Than A Weight
# Loss Advantage

### BY
### Ira Bowman

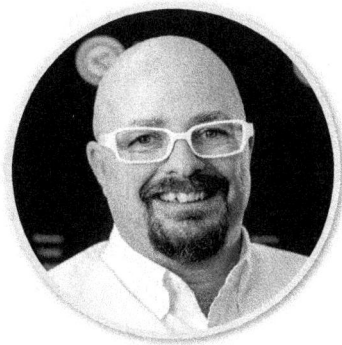

**Technique:** When I'm feeling a certain way, nothing is more helpful than a brisk walk. In fact, I went from averaging just under 3,000 steps a day to walking 20,000-25,000 steps per day simply because of the way it makes me feel and helps my mind work. I walk six or more times a day, up to 10,000 steps at a time, but more frequently, I walk shorter distances, like 2,000-5,000 steps at a time.

**How I discovered the technique:** I discovered this helpful technique by accident. I stumbled on this gem of a solution to my mental health struggles, and I'm so thankful I did. I was on a business trip for my photography business. Instead of renting a car or taking an Uber, on this particular three-day trip, I decided to walk everywhere except to the airport. The goal was to save money on the rides, but far more importantly, I discovered that it helped me clear my mind, reset my mental balance, and feel good from head to toe. When I got home, I adopted walking regularly into my daily routine. I initially aimed for 10,000 steps a day, six days a week, and one "power" day of 20,000 steps. However, I got hooked almost immediately on how walking made me feel and upped the daily goal to 20,000+ steps daily. I do cap it at 30,000, however, as the time it takes to walk me 30,000 is about four hours, which is simply too much time away from my home and family.

**How the technique helps me and how I use it regularly:** As I just mentioned, I started slowly, as my initial goal of 10,000 steps was not very aggressive; I simply wanted to get out daily and hit 10,000 steps a day. Why that number? I'm not exactly sure. It was four times what I had been averaging before this change. With COVID and working from home, I wasn't walking much. I sat at a computer most of the day, six days a week. I'd heard the number 10,000 tossed around on social media, so I figured it was as good as any other target. After about 30 days of implementing the new routine, I found it was not too hard to hit 20,000 steps a day, and I loved the benefits, so I ultimately upped my daily goal to hit that number.

Do I walk to be healthy? Yes, but not the healthy that most people think. Daily walking has helped me shed some pounds and loosen my clothes. Still, I'm doing it consistently because it helps me think, makes me happy, and provides me with a preventive medicine-like effect against depression and anger.

**Will walking daily help you?** I know that people come in all shapes and sizes. Similarly, I don't know if walking will have the same positive impact on your mindset as it does mine. Still, I love that this technique only costs time, so everyone can afford it, and it's as all-natural as you can get, without medication of any kind. If you are physically able to walk, I suggest you try it and find out for yourself. Like me, you might want to start with an easily achievable goal. My original goal was four times that of my normal step count, but you can adjust however you need, from two or three times or whatever seems manageable. If you get injured, give yourself a break, and you might want to consult with a physician, as I am not a doctor, nurse, or medical practitioner.

Right now, I walk about three hours every day. The time away from my desk in the sunshine and fresh (as fresh as we get in Southern California, anyway) air helps me think clearly, but I find myself working a bit along the way. I use my iPhone to take voice notes. I write comments on social media posts and even take client calls via phone or Zoom. As a business owner, having the freedom to set my schedule is nice, so this might not work for everyone.

I track my steps via the Health app on my iPhone, and I love seeing my weekly, monthly, and yearly progress as the averages keep increasing with each new month. The Health app is free, so the only cost involved with this new activity for me was about $40 on a good sun hat (that my kids laugh at), and I'm already on a new pair of shoes as my sneakers had worn out from the extra wear.

I've lost about 25 pounds in four months, which also helps my self-esteem. Here are the benefits of walking 10,000 or more steps a day from what I could find in my research online.

Walking over 10,000 steps a day is considered a significant achievement and has numerous benefits for your physical and mental well-being. Here are the top five benefits of walking over 10,000 steps a day:

1. Improved cardiovascular health: Walking is a great aerobic exercise that increases your heart rate and strengthens your cardiovascular system. Regularly achieving over 10,000 steps a day can help lower your risk of heart disease, improve blood circulation, and reduce blood pressure.

2. Weight management and increased calorie burn: Walking is a low-impact exercise that can aid in weight management. Walking over 10,000 steps daily helps burn extra calories, contributing to a calorie deficit and potential weight loss. It also boosts your metabolism, making it easier to maintain a healthy weight.

3. Enhanced mood and mental well-being: Physical activity, including walking, has been shown to positively impact mental health. Walking helps release endorphins, the feel-good hormones that can elevate your mood, reduce stress, and alleviate symptoms of anxiety and depression. Regular walking can also improve sleep quality and boost overall cognitive function.

4. Increased energy levels and stamina: Walking is a great way to boost your energy levels and combat fatigue. Regular physical activity, such as walking over 10,000 steps a day, can enhance your stamina, muscle strength, and endurance. As a result, you'll find yourself more capable of handling daily tasks and activities.

5. Joint and bone health: Walking is a low-impact exercise that puts less stress on your joints than higher-impact activities like running. Walking regularly and achieving over 10,000 steps a day can improve joint mobility,

strengthen muscles around the joints, and increase bone density. This can help prevent conditions like osteoporosis and reduce the risk of joint-related problems.

While walking over 10,000 steps a day is generally safe for most individuals, there are a few potential risks to consider:

1. Overuse injuries: Walking excessively without proper rest or recovery can lead to overuse injuries. Common examples include shin splints, stress fractures, and tendonitis. It's important to listen to your body, gradually increase your step count, wear appropriate footwear, and take rest days to allow your muscles and joints to recover.

2. Joint stress: While walking is a low-impact exercise, excessive walking can still stress your joints, particularly the knees and hips. Suppose you have existing joint conditions or injuries. In that case, it's essential to be mindful of your limits and consult a healthcare professional to ensure you're not putting undue strain on your joints.

3. Fatigue and burnout: Walking over 10,000 steps daily can be physically demanding, especially if you're not accustomed to high step counts. Pushing yourself too hard without adequate rest and recovery can lead to fatigue, burnout, and a higher risk of injuries. It's important to listen to your body, gradually increase your activity level, and prioritize rest days.

4. Neglecting other forms of exercise: Focusing solely on achieving 10,000 steps a day through walking may cause you to neglect other important components of fitness, such as strength training, flexibility, and cardiovascular exercises. Incorporating various exercises into your routine is beneficial to promote overall fitness and prevent muscle imbalances.

5. Risk of accidents and injuries: Walking outdoors or in unfamiliar environments may expose you to potential accidents or injuries, such as tripping, falling, or encountering hazardous conditions. Be mindful of your surroundings, wear appropriate footwear, and take necessary precautions to ensure your safety while walking.

Remember, while walking over 10,000 steps a day provides these benefits, listening to your body and gradually increasing your activity level if you're not already accustomed to high step counts is important. It's always recommended to consult with a healthcare professional before starting any new exercise routine.

On a personal note, walking has helped dramatically change my life for the good. My relationship with my wife and my children has improved. I was cranky, easily irritated, anxious, and generally unhappy. I spent far too much time in my office, sitting in front of my computer and working. I had low self-esteem and was way too overweight.

So, what changed? Walking helped me get a proper perspective on life. I'm sure a doctor can explain how the movement helps with the internal systems, but all I know is I was in a better mood, more friendly, and open to life away from my computer, and the change was dramatic. Strained relationships with my family started to heal and improve to the point where we're in a great place, maybe the best we've ever been.

I went from being unhappy most of the time to happy most of the time. I don't cringe when I look in the mirror anymore and have set new weight-related goals as the pounds continue to melt away, which doesn't hurt my feelings either.

I'm sharing all this because I always used to be anxious. I felt like I was slipping away. Walking wasn't a solution I was looking for, but I am so thankful I found it. If it can help any of you reading these words, I will be doubly happy to let you in behind the veneer I am so used to keeping. You know, the social media, "I'm great!" even when my world's falling apart. Why do we do that?

I know walking might not be the answer for everyone, or possibly even for most people, but I'm sure it can help some readers, which motivated me to share this story and technique. Frankly, it's the reason I asked my friends to join me in writing this book. I know they have different techniques for others to try, and I might try some of their techniques out myself.

What I hope everyone gets from this book is hope. You may or may not find the solution that works for you in this book; however, I believe there is a solution for all of us if we can keep an open mind and endure until we find the right one for us individually.

Some of you might wonder if there's ever a day I don't hit my goal. The answer is yes. I've missed the target goal a few times over the past four months, but thankfully, walking has now become part of my routine. My family, clients, and I know that I'm going to walk. I've met a lot of cool neighbors out there on the sidewalk and trails, too.

There's not much more important in life than our health. We only get one body, and it behooves us to do all we can to keep it physically, spiritually, and mentally healthy. I don't think I'll ever regret taking the time to invest in my mental health. I'm thankful that the process is also helping my body get back in shape. I encourage you to find the solution that works for you. I want nothing more than for you to be well and prosper fairly.

# Name Your Purpose and Tame Your Anxiety

## By
## Janet Hogan

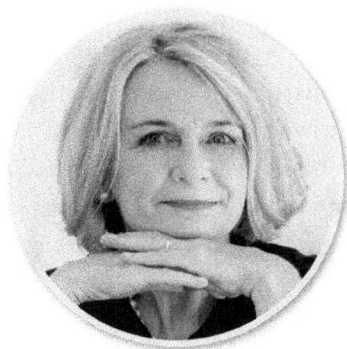

## Technique

When I feel overwhelmed and need clear direction, I refer to my Triangle of Success.

## My Tip

How often have you asked yourself, "Why am I here? What am I supposed to be doing with my life?" Discover freedom and clarity by bringing your life's purpose down to one simple word.

## How I Discovered This Technique

When I was around 11, one of my teachers confided to my mom that I had an "A" after my name. My mom puffed up, proud to have an A-grade student as her daughter.

"Oh, no," corrected my teacher. "What I mean is A for anxiety."

Like so many of us, I have carted around this unwelcome lodger for practically all my life. Like the fish in the fishbowl who can't see the murkiness of the water it's swimming in, I was largely unaware of the devastating effect of anxiety on my day-to-day quality of life.

After 25 years in business, I finally decided to hire a coach. The first thing he wanted to talk about was setting goals. Straight away, up came the familiar nervous clearing of my throat and pit in my stomach. The very word goal triggered all those shameful memories of New Year's resolutions brazenly made and never kept. Those five kilos I never lost. The $1 million I never made.

Then his eyes cornered mine, and he asked me the question I had never dared ask myself.

"Janet, what is it you really, *really* want?"

I gulped. To date, I'd devoted my whole life trying to make everybody else happy. What on earth did he even mean?

Then I felt that dreaded prickly sensation at the back of my eyes that comes just before they start welling up. *Please not now, don't break down at your very first session.*

I lamely shook my head.

"C'mon," he persisted. "There has to be *something* you want—something that excites you!"

I sat there, eyes glued to the wordless white sheet of paper staring back up at me, wishing for that one big golden goal to emerge.

But the harder I tried, the more blank the page became.

I sniffed, blew my nose, terrified the floodgates would open and reveal my terrible secret: I had no idea what I wanted. And worse, even if I did know, I felt I wouldn't have deserved it.

\* \* \*

Fast forward ten years, my husband Ralph and I did what many people do when they become bored with themselves; we moved—from Australia to Bali—searching for a change that would be as good as a permanent holiday.

We didn't know how long we would live on the Island of the Gods. The only way we could stay for an extended period was to set up our own company.

One of my favorite jobs in advertising was thinking up product names. I would lie in bed at night, mulling over the letters and syllables like monkey bars for my mind.

When creating a company in Bali came up, my immediate obsession was not who we speak to or can we even do it, but what will we call it.

While unpacking our umpteenth cardboard box, I found an old paperback, *In Tune with the Infinite* by Ralph Waldo Trine.

It was written back in 1897, the carefully crafted language reflecting the etiquette of the day.

As I scanned the parchment-colored pages, my eyes stopped at a word I'd never seen before. I couldn't work out what it meant, but I liked the sound of it and made a point of memorizing it before I fell asleep.

When I woke up the following day, Ralph sitting beside me, working on an essay, scribbling furiously on his notepad. Suddenly, he paused and looked up.

"Janno," he said, putting down his pen. "I need to pick your brain. There's a word I'm trying to remember from the days I read those Biggles adventure books as a kid. A word that means the toxic fog you'd see hanging over crocodile-infested swamps."

I didn't like being stumped on a word.

"Something to do with Hydrogen Sulfide?" I offered.

"No, no," said Ralph. "It's just one word."

"I dunno," I said. "But on another subject, I think I've found the name for our company."

"Fire away," said Ralph.

"How about we call it Miasma?"

Ralph turned and looked at me like he'd seen a poltergeist, then sprang backward out of the bed.

"My God, Janno, that's the word I was looking for!"

I shook my head, amazed. What were the chances? But then I slumped.

"We can't name our company after something that means toxic fog."

As it turned out, we had no choice. The word had chosen us. Very unsurprisingly, it was available, so we registered it.

That night, as I was thinking about the bizarre synchronicity of finding the word, I was taken back to that first session with my coach. When I wanted to think my way to what the real me wanted, I was overtaken by a kind of brain fog, a miasma of the mind that gave way to a paralyzing fear that kept me feeling stuck and confused.

Was this word miasma a spooky clue as to what I was supposed to be doing with my life? Was I perhaps meant to use my love of words honed from my 20 years in communications to help blow away that toxic fog of fear and help people find the confidence they needed to move forward?

What if I could take the exasperation I felt on that day with my coach and turn it into the inspiration to create a tool to give people instant clarity on what they truly want, who they truly are, an easy step-by-step process to discover where their brilliance lies?

So, I got to work.

Instead of a blank page, what would have helped me chart my way out of stuck-ness was a list of options, and not the usual carrots like the million in the bank, the red Ferrari in the garage, or the holiday on the Amalfi Coast, which provide an instant hit only to dissolve as quickly as cotton candy.

Nine times out of ten, what people think they want is only what their egoic mind tells them is the case.

*What if we changed the concept of goal setting from what our minds trick us into thinking we want to what our wiser, intuitive selves know we really need?*

I was looking for a way to finally quell the anxious self and fill that inner void, leading to a new state of peace, calm, freedom, and joy.

Through a process of elimination, which I narrowed to around 150 options, I developed a way to crystallize a person's real needs and potential for true happiness down to the most valuable trinity.

## YOUR THREE CORE NEEDS

I called this tool that emerged and changed my life the Triangle of Success.

And in case you're wondering how I define success, it's knowing what your true self wants and how to get it.

## HOW THE TECHNIQUE HELPS ME

When I took myself through the process and found my three core needs, I felt the relief of finally seeing in black and white what my true self had been yearning for.

Let me share my unique combo (yours will be different), so you understand how this works.

When I took myself through the Triangle of Success, here's what I came up with.

Core Need No. 3: Collaboration

Core Need No. 2: Impact

## Core Need No. 1: Prosperity

My third core need, collaboration, was a tap on both my shoulders from my true self. As an entrepreneur, I'd carried the weight of the world on those shoulders for way too long. I knew if I was going to make a serious dent in the world, I wouldn't do it as an army of one. It was time for this lone wolf to find her pack.

That would help me achieve my second core need: impact.

Impact was my heart saying to me:

*"Janet, enough playing small; you are here to make a difference. Time to haul yourself out of the chair of regret and start living the life you were born to live."*

I set my goal to positively impact 10,000 lives, knowing that at that point, I would have achieved the biggest prize of all, my first core need—prosperity.

Prosperity is my north star, my why. I had spent most of my 40 years in business believing I was as successful as the number of zeros in my bank account. Somehow, I had lost my true identity along the way.

It's estimated 80 percent of the working population is working to live, while only 20 percent live to work. As someone who has sacrificed most of my life on the altar of hard work, denying myself any real pleasure or satisfaction along the way, I know the pain of living as a human doing. This pain of self-betrayal fuels my passion for reversing those figures so that the 20 percent who love what they do become the 80 percent who currently don't.

Prosperity, for me, is a whole new way of looking at this thing we call a career, where our job transforms from being a mere occupation to a *pre*occupation that keeps us constantly engaged in life, where we have time to smell the roses, be engaging, funny, loving, and generous.

Put simply, prosperity means living in exchange, doing what I most enjoy, and being amply rewarded in the process.

I saw a pattern as I mapped out my Triangle and invited others to do the same. As it turned out, I'd lucked onto something extraordinary—a powerful formula.

The bottom two core needs, the third and second, are the elements you must master before claiming the prize at the top.

It's like a spiritual pathway—a personal formula for each of us to create the life we have always wanted but never knew how to attain.

I call this pathway your Golden Mission.

Here's what mine looks like:

*"Through collaboration and impact, I create a world of prosperity."*

As an ex-advertising veteran, I've written and read my share of forgettable corporate mission statements, the kind that gives you a warm, fuzzy feeling at the time and end up on the back of a toilet door.

But this mission statement was different. This was not a bunch of words about how to make a big corporation feel good about selling ice to Eskimos; this was about me, the person, the human brand.

The other great part was that with only three elements, even I could remember it.

As weeks passed into months, I shared the Triangle of Success with more people.

Then one day, I was listening to an interview with Simon Sinek, talking about how we need to focus on our why, not our what or how.

"That's all very fine," I said to myself. "But how do we know what our why, what, and how even are?"

And then the second penny dropped.

Here it was as clear as daylight.

If I could achieve my holy grail of prosperity—turning work into play—then the natural flow from that would be to want to teach others to do the same.

So, I realized that our core need is not just what our true self most wants; it's also what we have to give to others, our purpose—our why. Our greatest passion is formed from our ultimate pain.

The insights kept rolling in.

As for our what, the goal or tangible result we are here to achieve, that comes in the form of our second core need. Today, I teach entrepreneurs how to make their impact by getting clear on the problem they are uniquely placed to solve. Impact is that I bring to the table.

And finally, the third core need is our how.

Collaboration is how I make my impact and ultimately achieve prosperity. How am I doing this? By teaming up with like-minded people, fellow entrepreneurs in the mental wellness space who want to do well by doing good so we can support each other, leverage our respective audiences, and accelerate our journey in the most fun way possible.

## CAN THE TRIANGLE OF SUCCESS HELP YOU?

If, like me (and a few billion other folks), your anxious mind constantly worries about a future it cannot see, this simple tool gives shape to that uncertain future by introducing a destination that makes you feel good from the inside out.

Rewards we give ourselves that are externally derived may provide us with momentary joy, but they don't fill the void within. Once you fill that void, however, your anxious mind takes a back seat to your loving heart, which now has a tangible north star to follow.

Now that I've shared this tool with hundreds of people from all corners of the planet, I've discovered that no two combinations are the same. Like your thumbprint, your Golden Mission is unique to you.

So, will it work for you?

Well, here's what I know for sure.

Five years after creating this tool, I am still using it. In that time, my second and third core needs have changed in the same way your strategy and goals evolve as you do. But my why—my core need—has stayed the same.

In those five years, I have cleared the toxic fog of confusion, of not knowing what I was supposed to be doing with my life, so today, I am enjoying life from a place of clarity and confidence underpinned by an ever-present feeling of fulfillment.

The Triangle of Success helps me make sure that what I think about, talk about, and do are all aligned; in that space, I feel motivated and at peace simultaneously. My days of being stuck in a miasma of fear are long gone, and creating goals and strategies is now easy.

Hooray!

And hooray for you, too, if through your Triangle of Success, you unearth and follow your pathway to your ideal life.

If you would like to try out this tool for yourself, click here[1]

It's free; it's easy to do, and we'll even email you a short explanation about your results.

One final reminder: Your Triangle of Success is a clear instruction from your true self to you. Take it seriously. I have my Triangle pinned up to my wall and look at it daily. I encourage you to do the same.

As a confessed word nerd, I'd like to finish with one of my favorite quotes.

"In the beginning was the Word, and the Word was God."

If God lives inside of you, it is undoubtedly within your heart. This neat little tool is a simple way to leave your thinking mind behind and connect with your loving heart. Before you begin, find a quiet place. Become present. And be open to receiving whatever magical word your heart whispers back to you.

# Transforming Traumatized Children— And How to Use This Knowledge to Transform Yourself

BY
DR. DAVID FOSTER

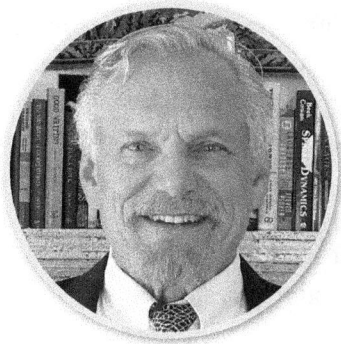

Have you ever had a dream so bizarrely vivid and surreal that it felt like a different reality? I invite you to enter my real-life experience, which felt just as dreamlike. This journey might be challenging, and the story might shift, just like in a dream.

As if you're in a scene from a Kafka novel, you find yourself trapped inside a plexiglass cage with a serial killer. The surreal surroundings feel like a massive energy sink, draining all hope. How in the world did you end up here? You recall entering this place, but now, you're locked in this bizarre enclosure.

You remember the sequence of events that led you here: It felt like stepping into a horror movie with a daunting castle-like structure with armed guards. You were led to a steel door with a small spy window. Once identified, you stepped into a small chamber and heard the door shut behind you, the sound of a heavy key turning the lock echoing in your ears.

After securing the first door, the second door was unbolted and unlocked. You entered a sterile area where visitors waited as if in suspended animation. You were led through another locked door, down a hallway, and through another locked door into a room with a plexiglass cage. You entered this cage and heard the door locked behind you. There, you came face-to-face with the first serial killer you've ever met, a man with a mustache and shaggy dark hair, staring at you with dark, lifeless eyes.

Fast forward: You are sitting with a seven-year-old boy, placed in the highest level of residential care because he threatened his new foster parents with a butcher knife. He can't stop bouncing on his cushioned chair and blurting out impulsive random observations. When you try to connect with him, he responds with anger and defiance. As you review his history, you can't help but notice the similarities with the serial killer you met in the plexiglass cage.

What do the serial killer and the seven-year-old boy have in common? They both had parents who were addicted, neglected them, and severely abused them. They were left in places that couldn't handle their wild behaviors or, in the case of the murderer, where he was further tortured and molested.

The path that led me to these encounters was not one I had planned or desired. But along this unexpected journey, I learned a great deal about how devastating the effects of childhood abuse and neglect can be.

Some of you reading this might know firsthand the crippling effects of childhood trauma and the anxiety disorder called Post Traumatic Stress Disorder (PTSD). For all of us, the costs are immense, and the benefits of effective interventions can be life changing. Once we understand the economic, social, psychological, and physical costs, and sometimes even deadly outcomes, it becomes clear why we must find effective interventions to prevent these outcomes. Wouldn't you agree?

The economic costs alone are staggering, not to mention the incalculable cost of human suffering and loss. In the US, state child welfare costs for the fiscal year 2018 were $33 billion.[1] Additionally, research-based estimates conservatively put the lifetime cost per child after they age out of the system at $210,012 to over $600,000.[2] For those who have failed mul-

---

[1]   Child Welfare: Purposes, Federal Programs, and Funding, Congressional Research Services, January 13, 2023. Almost half of these costs are for foster care and other out-of-home placements, primarily due to severe abuse and neglect, or factors that make a parent unable to care for their child, like incarceration, disabling mental illness, or addiction. With long-term care, not only does the yearly cost per child rise, but the lifetime cost increases as well.

[2]   The Unseen Costs of Foster Care: A Social Return on Investment Study; www.allainnovations.org. This is probably a significant underestimate, since medical costs alone for this population is astounding. A Kaiser study, for example, found that that the most expensive utilizers of care were the severely abused. (The Relation Between Adverse Childhood Experiences and Adult Health: *Turning Gold into Lead,* Perm J. 2002 Winter; 6(1):

tiple placements or are unmanageable at other levels of care, the cost is $75,000 per year, and the lifetime costs skyrocket.

But what if we have methods that can change the life path of traumatized and neglected children, and these interventions save not just dollars but, more importantly, redeem human potential? Shouldn't we implement them immediately? If these methods can work for complex, deep-end cases of highly traumatized, at-risk children—and we are convinced they do—then many of them can be applied by any person living with PTSD in their daily life, including you.

Childhood abuse and neglect affect every level of life—biological, psychological, social, moral, and spiritual. Therefore, an integrated approach to transforming these issues is required.

The brain and nervous system that integrate the body can be likened to a computer's hardware.[3] If the hardware is damaged in some way, the computer malfunctions. Our social and experiential programming can be compared to the software that encodes in brain pathways as implicit and explicit memories and our internal representational systems of self, other, and world.

The energy that animates us and the electromagnetic features of the body that every cell produces, which collectively envelope us and can be accessed to heal or damage us, is like the

---

44–47; https://nhttac.acf.hhs.gov/soar/eguide/stop/adverse_childhood_experiences.  put the medical costs at $210,012

[3]  Like any analogy or metaphor it is not entirely accurate and, in some ways misleading. One example is that in the brain the programming (software) effects the  brain structure and processes, and vice versa, but this is not true in our current computers. Nonetheless, the computer analogy will be helpful in understanding the various levels of our interventions.

electricity needed to awaken the computer. Without power, the computer is dead or asleep and nonfunctional.[4]

When one has suffered repeated abuse or neglect, dramatic changes occur in the brain, body, programmed memory, and behavioral circuits. Behavior originates in the brain, which, as the organ of the mind, impacts our learning, thinking, and emotional states. The changes abuse causes in the child's neurology increases the odds that they will develop difficulties learning and often truncates their potential with handicapping and disempowering limiting beliefs and negative emotions. It can even alter one's physiology and behavioral responses at the epigenetic or transgenerational level, biologically and behaviorally passing on limited resilience and behavioral flexibility. The traumas are frequently re-lived, and protective, sympathetic nervous system freeze-flight-fight responses are easily triggered at inappropriate times and ways.

Without help in resolving these problems, adequate education, and models of alternative behaviors, the cycle of abuse is frequently passed on from generation to generation.

---

[4]    In ancient traditions, these three aspects, hardware, software, energy source, are referred to as body, soul, and spirit.. We are beginning to understand that some ancient traditions seemed to know how to operate on the energetic/spiritual or quantum level of reality. At this level, the laws of Newtonian physics are transcended and one can enter the "woo" realm of quantum physics. Mastering the principles at this level can lead to remarkably rapid changes that sometimes seem magical, but are completely lawful at the quantum level. Scientific attempts at describing the science of operating at this level has been bravely done by, among others, Dr. Larry Farwell in his books *How Consciousness Commands Matter* and *The Science of Creating Miracles*.

When we have intervened in the multigenerational cycle of abuse with motivated parents, in conjunction with Child Protective Services, and when they are given the appropriate treatments for their addictions and mental illnesses, provided trauma resolution interventions that resolve their traumas, and taught life skills and parenting tools, we can often prevent their children from long-term out-of-home placement and the accompanying traumas this can cause.

But this is not always possible, and we must help the child for whom reunification is not possible and, most challenging, for those who have failed multiple placements.

Due to the advances in neuroscience and brain imaging, we have a much more sophisticated understanding of brain-behavior relationships and more tools for assisting the brain in its self-healing and self-regulation. As noted above, we know how early childhood neglect and abuse and even failure of parent-child attunement can affect the developing brain, alter its structure, and destabilize brain physiology. Concurrently, there have been significant advances in medical and non-medical methods for stabilizing the brain. There has also been remarkable progress in trauma resolution therapies. And we know so much more about the developing brain and mind[5] and how to nurture and coach it to become the amazing creative power it can potentially become.

So, what does an integrated, innovative approach for traumatized children look like? The following sequence of interventions presupposes that two vital factors are present: rapport and trustworthy competence.

---

[5]    See, for example, Daniel Segal's excellent book *The Developing Mind*.

With rapport and trust established, the first step is a physical[6] and neurological evaluation, a comprehensive psycho-social history, and a psychiatric/psychological evaluation. We also vigorously promote the beneficial effects of exercise, a healthy diet, good sleep hygiene, and, if needed, supplements like vitamin D3.[7] So, consult with your nutritionally informed healthcare professional about testing for these and adding appropriate supplements.

We also find the quantitative electroencephalogram (QEEG) to be a very useful evaluation tool in making treatment decisions about how best to stabilize the brain.[8]

---

[6] Blood work to evaluate for metabolic and nutritional issues including thyroid, and nutritional deficiencies such as iodine, vitamin D3, Folate and B12 deficiencies. We also find it useful to test for MTHFR DNA mutations. Many Americans are Vitamin D3 deficient, which is necessary for serotonin production, and therefore, can be a cause of anxiety and depression. This can be remedied by D3 replacement. Up to 60% of those with anxiety and depression have an MTHFR genetic mutation, which can be remedied with methyl folate replacement. Low iodine can lead to false readings of thyroid levels, and if low, can remedy hypothyroidism which can cause depression.

[7] All of these interventions can apply to anyone who is depressed or anxious.

[8] Despite some controversy, we find convincing evidence in the research, and even more convincing evidence in our clinical work for the cost-effective value of the QEEG in both medication selection and in mapping out neurofeedback interventions. In our experience, it is even more useful and cost effective than brain imaging studies like SPECT and PET scans. The QEEG is a standard electroencephalogram (EEG) measuring brain waves. We then send this data to a center in the Netherlands that uses sophisticated computer analysis that compares it to

The next step is brain stabilization; without it, one is unlikely to succeed in the following interventions. Brain stabilization in seriously traumatized children and adolescents can help prevent more serious psychiatric problems in adulthood.[9]

Without brain calming and stabilization, it is more challenging to teach self-soothing behaviors like mindfulness meditation, yoga, and specific breathing techniques or induce motivation

---

norms and to thousands of other age matched eegs and to other brain studies, like functional MRIs to give a sophisticated statistically significant comparison to what other brain studies would look like, had they been done. In particular, the brain wave ratios tell us a great deal about which medications are most likely to help and what brainwave training might render the most optimal brain functioning. For example, ADHD can have multiple causes and differences in brain wave ratios. The "garden variety" ADHD has too many slow (sleep) wave activity relative to focussed (beta wave) activity. This version responds best to stimulants which "wake the brain up." Too many high alpha or high beta waves respond to different medications better and to different neurofeedback training.

[9] It is rare, in my experience, to find an adult with complex childhood onset PTSD who does display, at the least, Bipolar II or Bipolar III symptoms – even without a family history of bipolar disorder. This is because complex child trauma damages, among other areas, the same brain structures involved in bipolar disorder. And, they respond to the same best practice interventions for bipolar disorders. The unstable PTSD brain frequently does not experience the activated (manic or hypomanic) states as euphoria, but rather, agitation, anxiety or panic, or agitation and irritability. The worst is what is called a mixed state often experienced as agitation and depression at the same time or in rapid cycling patterns. This usually requires expert medical/psychiatric intervention.

for exercise and healthy nutrition. With brain optimization, these non-medical practices become essential ingredients in managing the symptoms of PTSD.[10]

Brain stabilization is followed by resourcing methods,[11] which can rapidly create the internal representations of nurturing and limiting figures needed for self-support and self-regulation. This is then complemented by teaching life skills.[12]

Once these interventions are successful, we can begin effective trauma and grief[13] resolution therapies.

When traumatic memories are no longer activated, teaching and coaching to learn how to use the directives of the unconscious mind in formatting goals and learning the steps and actions required for the creation of desired outcomes, including how to overcome resistances—limiting beliefs, negative emotions, etc.—to achieve any truly desired goal.

---

[10] As Ira Bowman points out in his chapter, exercise is key, and, as the research shows, perhaps the single most important factor in regulating anxiety and mood.

[11] See for example Philip Mansfield's book *Dyadic Resourcing: Creating a Foundation for Processing Trauma (Excellence in EMDR Therapy)*, CreateSpace Independent Publishing Platform (August 26, 2010).

[12] 6 of these life skills are described in the book *The Solution*, Laurel Mellin; Harper Collins, 1996.and include learning self-nurturing and self-limit setting, body pride, good health, balanced eating and mastery pride. I highly recommend reading it. Also important is increasing social support, like ACA, etc.

[13] See the work of Robert Pynoos, et al. Specifically, *Trauma and Grief Component Therapy for Adolescents: A Modular Approach to Treating Traumatized and Bereaved Youth*, Saltzman, Layne, Pynoos, et al. Cambridge University Press; 1st edition (January 12, 2018).

Availability to supervise and educate the caretakers, where needed, and support the structures or holding environments that support the changes that these interventions facilitate can be another key component to success. So, for example, parenting classes may be needed to enable reuniting with parents, assisting foster parents in managing difficult behaviors,[14] or in group homes, supporting and interdigitating with the clear routines and structures and appropriate behavioral rewards and clear, kind, firm limits. Supervising and providing education to staff that helps them better understand and appropriately support children under their care can significantly enhance the desired changes.

Now, let's look at the individual interventions in more detail to see how they are applied.

Brain stabilization is required because these highly traumatized children and adults have over-aroused sympathetic freeze-flight-fight systems with a brain that did not develop the brain structures and neural pathways that grow in nurturing and soothing parent-child interactions that accompany the internalizing of the emotional mirroring and soothing needed to develop a child's right hemisphere frontal inhibition and self-soothing parasympathetic pathways.[15]

Brain stabilization impacts the hardware and makes the needed changes in the software possible. It can be likened to installing

---

[14]   For excellent ways to do this read *The Connected Child: Bring Hope and Healing to Your Adoptive Family*, by Wendy Lyons Sunshine, et al., McGraw Hill; 1st edition (April 22, 2007).

[15]   This is often complicated by damage to the brain caused by exposure in utero to toxins like alcohol and other drugs. See also Allan Schore's Affect Regulation and the *Origin of the Self: The Neurobiology of Emotional Development* (Psychology Press & Routledge Classic Editions).

electrical surge protection to prevent the hardware from being damaged and enable repair while the computer runs. So, also do the non-medical interventions like proper nutrition, exercise, breathing, meditation practices, etc.

In our experience, getting these very unstable, traumatized brains to the place where these children can learn self-soothing and self-regulation almost always requires the judicious use of medication followed by neurofeedback. Without these interventions to stabilize and optimize brain functioning, it is challenging to generalize learning of self-soothing behaviors like breathing, time outs, and new, more realistic cognitive evaluations to determine safety, value, and control. With the added support of neuro-biofeedback, one can often eventually reduce or even eliminate the need for medication.[16]

Without medication, these very traumatized children and adolescents are much less likely to efficiently benefit from neurofeedback and interventions to resolve their PTSD or to maintain stable forever home placements. Additionally, when there is a family history of severe mental illness, as symptoms and signs emerge in the child, the appropriate use of medications can prevent or attenuate the development of these mental illnesses.

Neurofeedback or neuro-biofeedback is a crucial ingredient in our integrative approach. Neurofeedback is a non-invasive form of biofeedback that reinforces the brain's ability to find

---

[16] Some readers may be tempted to throw the baby out with the bath water, at this juncture, because of their experience or concern about the overuse or inappropriate use of medication. While it is true that medications have been overused, and even inappropriately used, the judicious and knowledgeable use of appropriate medication is often the only way, in our experience at this time, to achieve brain stabilization.

brainwave patterns that enable the brain to heal itself and self-regulate. One can then choose appropriate brain wave states, like focus or relaxation.

Once the brain is stabilized, trauma resolution therapies integrating Cognitive Behavioral Therapy (CBT), Exposure Therapy, Eye Movement Desensitization and Reprocessing (EMDR)—especially EMDR 2.0—Flash, Timeline Therapy,[17] and Brainspotting can be applied. A well-trained therapist is required to implement these therapies effectively.

The next step, when desired, is coaching in life skills and learning to operate one's brain and mind. When one understands the behavioral neurology of classical Pavlovian conditioning and how to anchor desired states of mind and behaviors—as all optimal performers in every field from sports to politics do—and operant Skinnerian conditioning and how to reinforce desired behaviors in oneself positively, you have a significant leg up on controlling your brain states and behavior. Therefore, you are more likely to create the outcomes you want.

What can you do if you were traumatized?

Start by finding competent professional help. You're set to change when you can identify the original trauma and the root limiting belief and a realistic empowering belief to replace it.

In all effective interventions, there are four steps. With competent, supportive supervision, you can use them to transmute the traumas.

---

[17] A researched for of Timeline Therapy (Mental and Emotional Release or MER) in moderately to severely impaired adults on psychiatric medications, found, in five year follow-up, that 90% had no recurrance of their symptoms <u>and</u> were on no medications.

Step one is the hardest. It is identifying the sensory memory of the trauma and its accompanying limiting belief and activating the emotional responses the trauma memories trigger; the more intensely, the better. Since this is often happening randomly, why not dive into it? But don't do this unless you have supportive internal and external resources like trustworthy, competent people and a safe place, both in your imagination and in your external environment, to which you can retreat whenever you need. When activated, the trauma memory is using your working memory, which must be lit up as intensely as possible so that your unconscious mind can process it with minimal distress in the next step.

When one understands how to activate the circuits of belief and their accompanying emotions, one can uproot dysfunctional belief circuits and reprogram the brain with more functional beliefs. Our belief systems (software) about ourselves and the world can empower us or limit us. When one is traumatized, it is usual for powerful limiting beliefs to control our behavior.[18] Effective trauma resolution therapies can profoundly influence this level.

The next step is breaking the activated trauma circuit through distraction, like refocusing on some real sensory experience in the present—literally coming to your senses.[19] Another option is to try patterned alternating movements, such as back-and-forth eye movement, running in place, dance moves, etc. This breaks the working memory circuit and allows your brain to begin to process the trauma unconsciously and rap-

---

[18]   For example, the beliefs that I am not safe, I am not valued, I am helpless, I'm not enough, I'm defective or dirty, etc. can be very disempowering and also cause self-fulfilling dysfunctional patterns of behavior.

[19]   Having mint or lavender oils to smell, noticing the colors and sounds in your environment, feeling your shoes in your feet, etc.

idly without conscious interference. Once you have lit up the traumatic memory, try to distract yourself for 15 minutes, even if, at first, you can only do it for 15 seconds.

Next is connecting to the internal and external resources currently accessible to you that would have enabled you to feel safe, valued, in control, etc. This can be as simple as recognizing that you survived and are a survivor, not a victim, or imagining having the help you needed or would provide yourself now. Surprisingly, it often helps the most if the resource you internalize is a fictional character who can provide the safety, sense of value or control, or gives the positive message or belief you need instead of the limiting beliefs usually associated with trauma. This is where the dyadic resourcing done by a trained therapist can be very powerful.[20]

The last step is to imagine using your newfound resourcefulness and resources when confronted in the future with events or circumstances that previously triggered your traumatic responses.

Taking care of yourself is the most significant contribution you can make. When you are whole and know how to manage your issues, you can be more beneficial to others, even if only as a model of how to create a happy, productive life. This is far more important in impacting the world than many believe.

What's next?

There are amazing researchers and clinicians worldwide who are working to decrease the causes and consequences of child trauma. What if, in collaboration, small, highly successful pilot projects could be replicated and applied anywhere to transform children, youth, and their caretakers in all Child Welfare and Juvenile Justice Systems? What if, since it demonstrably

---

[20]   Ibid Philip Manfield

reduces long-term costs at every level and helps the most at risk, it is applied to all who want and need it? You would do what you could to support it, wouldn't you?

As for the oppositional, defiant, distractible, impulsive, highly traumatized, and emotionally labile seven-year-old, he is now nine and still benefiting from the interventions described above. He is happily stable, excelling at school, and no longer troubled by his traumatic early life. Best of all, he is eagerly "all in" as he is beginning a new life with an amazing "forever family."

And the murderer in the Plexiglass cage? His name was William Bonin, the infamous Freeway Killer who murdered a minimum of twenty-one young men and boys. I spent three consecutive days in that cage with him, doing a neuropsychiatric evaluation and pondering what could possibly cause such devastating outcomes. What was in the mind of this monster?

Every evening, I attempted to reconstruct his development by reviewing stacks of historical records from his past, including child protective services, descriptions of his family, mental health and health records, records from his orphanage placement, school and juvenile justice placements, military records and prior prison records where he was incarcerated for sexual assaults on minors, and declarations of those who knew him in various placements and schools.

When I finally put the pieces in place, it was devastating to retrospectively see all the missed opportunities that might have prevented the tragic outcomes. Even more difficult was when I experienced making the "phenomenological reduction" and "got into his head" and experienced his vengeful, twisted longing for someone to understand what his childhood experiences of helplessness and terror were like and to be able to possess them forever, without the betrayals like those who testified against him, resulting in prior imprisonments.

Being the first of dozens of subsequent death row evaluations, I took weeks to recover from my encounters with Bonin. At a cost of approximately 12 million dollars for death row placement and the appeals process, Bill Bonin was executed by lethal injection on San Quentin's Death Row. My experience with him has greatly motivated me to help create better outcomes for traumatized children.

# Take the Edge Off Stress with Ha Breathing from Hawai'i

BY
ERIC ROSEN

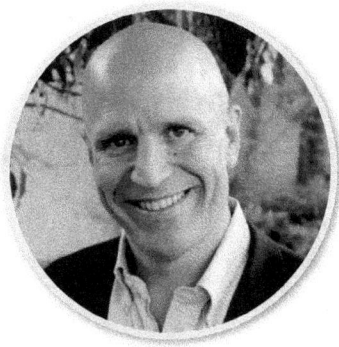

Like many of us, Evan had to pivot and start working from home when the county he lived and worked in entered lockdown. As a senior manager, he would walk around and get a read on how things were going by engaging his team members face-to-face in different areas of the building. To partially make up for this, he found himself scheduling more Zoom meetings, but this new way of working lacked those friendly and impromptu occasions to glean insights that were a hall-mark of his management style. Apart from our health concerns back then, Evan's inability to keep his finger on the pulse of his department in the way he had been accustomed to added yet another layer of stress for him.

As the founder of a Silicon Valley startup (and an avid med-itator), Maryam had to deliver more than her fair share of pitches to potential investors. Even though she has deep tech-nical knowledge, is well-spoken, and is altogether presentable, this was a very real source of stress for her. When it became necessary to shift to Zoom, she thought it would alleviate her fear of public speaking; however, the inability to read body language and the room's energy over video left her feeling no less anxious. And then, one day, it dawned on her. *Why not weave what I know from meditation and breathwork into my presentation activities?* But how?

## WHAT IS HA BREATHING?

Ha breathing comes from Ancient Hawai'i. It is a simple and effective way to take the edge off of stress. Ha means breath in Hawai'ian, and it's the first syllable in Hawai'i. Hawai'i translated means "Supreme life force that rides on the breath."

### Why Do Ha Breathing?

In today's hectic world, it's a fair bet we can all benefit from a tool for relieving stress that can easily be adapted for use in both public and private settings. As you'll soon see, the flexible nature of Ha breathing makes it convenient and practical to incorporate into your daily life anytime, anywhere.

When I work with clients one-on-one in my coaching and hypnosis practice, I walk them through Ha breathing at the start of Session 1. Ha becomes a foundational piece of everything we do from then on in terms of habit-breaking, guided visualization, goal setting, emotional baggage release, belief change, and more.

What Exactly is It?

When Ha breathing, we breathe in for a count of four through the nostrils and exhale out of the mouth for a count of eight. This exhale out of the mouth that is double the length of the inhale through the nose is a defining feature of Ha breathing. Pushing more air out than we breathe in will ease us into the calm of our parasympathetic nervous system.

According to the Cleveland Clinic[1], the parasympathetic nervous system helps relax you in calm times and balances your body's short-term survival responses.

If you cannot maintain the four seconds in and eight seconds out breathing pattern (a total of 12 seconds), it's okay to go with a shorter total duration. For example, three seconds in and six seconds out. Simply keep this one-to-two ratio.

An overlooked benefit of regularly doing Ha breathing is that it promotes diaphragmatic breathing. Many people tend to breathe through the mouth rather than originating the breath from their diaphragms. Breathing through the mouth all the time, including when you're sleeping, can lead to problems.

Mouth breathing can cause crooked teeth, facial deformities, or poor growth in children. In adults, chronic mouth breathing can cause bad breath and gum disease. It can also worsen

---

[1]    Parasympathetic Nervous System (PSNS) https://my.cleveland clinic.org/health/body/23266-parasympathetic-nervous-system-psns

symptoms of other illnesses.[2] Mouth breathing leads to dry mouth, which means there is not much saliva in your mouth, which can wash the bacteria from the mouth, which causes the bacteria to grow on the tongue and results in bad breath.[3]

Breathing from the diaphragm has various benefits that can affect your entire body. As such, it is common to many meditation and relaxation techniques, which can lower your stress levels, lower your blood pressure, and regulate other critical bodily processes.[4]

One of the biggest benefits of diaphragmatic breathing is reducing stress. Being stressed keeps your immune system from working at full capacity. This can make you more susceptible to numerous conditions. Over time, long-term or chronic stress—even from seemingly minor inconveniences like traffic—can sometimes lead to anxiety or depression.[5]

While Ha breathing is altogether simple to understand and do, I thought it would be even more helpful to my clients if I provided them with a means to measure its effectiveness at the moment. In the context of our work, feeling more relaxed from the start in a quantifiable way (with an easy technique they can do on their own) nurtures the belief that more positive changes are to come. Since our beliefs tend to make for self-fulfilling prophecies, you can see how important Ha

---

[2]   What to Know About Mouth Breathing https://www.healthline.com/health/mouth-breathing

[3]   Why Mouth Breathing Is Bad & How To Stop It In 5 Ways https://missionmeditation.com/why-mouth-breathing-is-bad/

[4]   What Is Diaphragmatic Breathing? https://www.healthline.com/health/diaphragmatic-breathing

[5]   What Is Diaphragmatic Breathing? https://www.healthline.com/health/diaphragmatic-breathing

breathing plays in helping them achieve the results they seek. As the old expression goes, "Everything begins with the breath."

To further aid my clients' success, it is important that they not only get immediate and measurable benefits from Ha breathing but also view it as easy to do on their own in any environment, whether it's a high-stakes business meeting, a tense family moment, or travel to places unknown. For this reason, in addition to including measurements with Ha breathing, I added variations to Ha breathing itself. These variations give my clients options on how they can weave Ha breathing into whatever situation they find themselves in. Knowing the quick results they've already achieved are reproducible in various circumstances, they begin to feel empowered in their lives.

Here are the four Ha Breathing variations. The third and fourth variations blend Hawai'ian Ha breathing with yogic Ujjayi breathing from India. Ujjayi creates a nice ocean sound in your throat that only you are likely to hear.

| Variation # | Description |
|---|---|
| 1 | Eyes open. Inhale for four seconds; exhale for eight seconds. |
| 2 | Eyes closed. Inhale for four seconds; exhale for eight seconds. |
| 3 | Eyes closed. Inhale for four seconds; exhale out of the mouth with mouth closed for eight seconds. |
| 4 | Eyes open. Inhale for four seconds; exhale out of the mouth with mouth closed for eight seconds. |

We will discuss how you can do Ha breathing with measurement and the four variations later in this chapter. Here is a brief overview of the process I do with my clients:

- They gauge their current free-floating stress or tension level on a scale of 0 to 10, so we have a baseline.
- I walk them through Variation #1 of Ha breathing.
- We measure their stress level again. (Usually, it drops to a lower number.)
- We do Variation #2 (the same as #1 but with eyes closed as a slight modification).
- We measure again, and it drops a little more.
- We do Variation #3 (the same as #2 but with the mouth closed while exhaling out of the mouth).
- We measure again, and typically, the number reaches a new low.
- We do Variation #4 (the same as #3 but with eyes open).
- We measure again.

The final measurement tends to be quite low and possibly zero if it hasn't gone there already.

Even if we don't get to zero but the client sees the number is significantly lower than before they started Ha breathing, it sets them up well to do the deeper work that follows (i.e., dumping their emotional baggage and ditching their limiting beliefs).

## HOW TO DO HA BREATHING, STEP BY STEP

Now, let's dive into how you can do Ha breathing independently. Remember that with any variations involving eye closure, you want to be in a place where it is safe to do so.

If you are doing Ha Breathing for the first time and would like to replicate the initial in-session approach (which includes measurements of your stress or tension before and after each variation), follow these steps:

| Step # | Measurement | Variation | Description |
|--------|-------------|-----------|-------------|
| 1 | Baseline | | Gauge your current free-floating stress or tension level on a scale of 0 to 10, where 10 is maximum intensity, and 0 means none. |
| 2 | | 1st | Eyes open. Inhale for four seconds; exhale for eight seconds. Do four rounds. |
| 3 | After 1st Variation | | Gauge your current free-floating stress or tension level on a scale of 0 to 10 and notice the new, lower level (in all likelihood). |
| 4 | | 2nd | Eyes closed. Inhale for four seconds; exhale for eight seconds. Do four rounds. |
| 5 | After 2nd Variation | | Gauge your current free-floating stress or tension level on a scale of 0 to 10. Notice how it compares with previous readings |

| | | | |
|---|---|---|---|
| 6 | | 3rd | Eyes closed. Inhale for four seconds; exhale out of the mouth with mouth closed for eight seconds (notice the ocean-like sound). Do four rounds. |
| 7 | After 3rd Variation | | Gauge your current free-floating stress or tension level on a scale of 0 to 10. Notice how it compares with previous readings |
| 8 | | 4th | Eyes open. Inhale for four seconds; exhale out the mouth with mouth closed for eight seconds (notice the ocean-like sound). Do four rounds. |
| 9 | After 4th Variation | | Gauge your current free-floating stress or tension level on a scale of 0 to 10. Notice how it compares with previous readings. |

# COMMON QUESTIONS ABOUT HA BREATHING

Here are some commonly asked questions about Ha breathing so you can incorporate it into your everyday life with a clear vision of what it can and cannot do. This will help you get the most out of it.

Q. Will Ha breathing enable me to release my negative emotions and limiting beliefs?

A. As we enter the calm of the parasympathetic nervous system with Ha breathing, exiting our existing thought patterns becomes much easier. In the process, our capacity to welcome different perspectives and derive new meanings from our lives' events, relationships, and patterns expands.

Is clearing negative emotions and limiting beliefs a given with Ha breathing? While not out of the question, to make such a claim outright would be a stretch. The same could be said of meditation. Neither technique is designed to release negative emotions and limiting beliefs; however, they serve as an excellent prelude to other methods like Mental and Emotional Release® that are effective at bringing us to a better emotional constitution and belief structure.

Nevertheless, there are myriad ways in which breathwork and meditation are beneficial to us. I liken them to hygiene for the nervous system. We brush our teeth every day for our oral hygiene, so why not meditate or do Ha breathing every day to benefit our nervous systems?

Q. Can Ha breathing have any negative side effects?

A. Ha breathing is considered safe for healthy people as it does not focus on breath retention or fast breathing, which could be an issue for people with high blood pressure. Likewise, Ha is not forceful with the breath, which might not be suitable for people with heart disease. If you have any concerns with Ha or other breathing techniques, it is best to consult your doctor first.

Q. Do you recommend certain variations of Ha breathing for particular circumstances?

A. Yes. Variations #2 and #3 are the ones my clients enjoy the most when in session. This is because they are closed-eye techniques, and eye closure promotes greater relaxation and better preparation for our change work. Variations #1 and #4 come in handy when you are among people and want to ease your way out of stress without anyone knowing you are doing something. This is especially the case with Variation #4, as having eyes open and mouth closed is the approach my clients find to be the most discreet.

## EPILOGUE

Getting back to Maryam, we met through mutual friends. As she shared her experience with me, I had her try out Ha breathing. The Ujjayi variations of Ha breathing were familiar to her since she was a meditator and yogi, after all.

She now had the answer she was looking for. She would do Ha breathing before and after hopping on Zoom because she could do Variation #2 with eyes closed and mouth open (for the most relaxing effect). Any time during conversations with investors where she wasn't doing the talking, she would ease into Variation #4 with eyes open and mouth closed (to remain calm without calling undue attention to herself).

The more she blended these variations into her business day, the more those old worries about body language and room energy faded. And, as I understand it, her company is faring better on the funding front.

When the stress started getting too edgy for him, Evan found me online and reached out. At that time, I, like him, also pivoted to an all-virtual practice. Before we got into the deeper work of clearing out his negative thoughts and dissolving the self-beat-up he had been putting himself through since he was a kid, I taught Evan Ha breathing. He got the hang of it right away.

At the start of our next session, he shared with me that his knee-jerk tendency to schedule yet another Zoom call had abated. He attributed this to the clear mind Ha breathing gives him. This, in turn, revealed to Evan other ways of raising the productivity of his teams.

For some, Ha breathing can be a real game changer. For others, it serves as an ideal gateway into deeper transformational work. Either way, it can lead you to a more empowered life. Enjoy.

| Readability Statistics | ? | X |
|---|---|---|
| **Counts** | | |
| Words | | 2,274 |
| Characters | | 11,435 |
| Paragraphs | | 93 |
| Sentences | | 136 |
| **Averages** | | |
| Sentences per Paragraph | | 2.5 |
| Words per Sentence | | 15.8 |
| Characters per Word | | 4.6 |
| **Readability** | | |
| Flesch Reading Ease | | 63.1 |
| Flesch-Kincaid Grade Level | | 8.1 |
| Passive Sentences | | 2.2% |
| | OK | |

# TIP:
# THE RECIPE FOR RESILIENCE

### BY
### JIM LOMOT

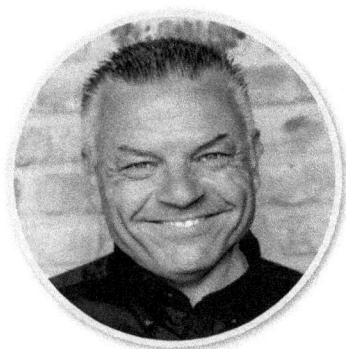

*"Your big opportunity may be where you are right now."*

-Napoleon Hill

Perhaps you aren't feeling very good about where you are in your life right now. Maybe you're feeling frustrated. You might feel lost and unsure about what direction to even go anymore. Is there a habit or addiction that has power over you? Have you experienced a significant loss? Do you feel alone? Are you at the end of your rope and feeling hopeless?

If this sounds like you, I'm so glad you're reading this right now. Look, I'm not a doctor or a therapist. And, truth be told, the other authors in this book are probably more professionally trained than me. But here's what I know: I have sat exactly where you're sitting now. I have been right where you are at this moment. I have felt frustrated with life. I have felt lost and unsure of the next step. I have felt powerless against destructive habits and addictions. I have experienced significant loss. I have felt alone and misunderstood. Worst of all, I have felt hopeless.

However, I have good news. I have overcome all these things.

And the great news is that you can, too!

You might be asking, how did I overcome these things? In a word: *resilience*. My goal for the rest of this chapter is to tell you a story. The story will share the "Everyday Techniques to Overcome Anxiety and Mental Health Struggles" that I used to develop unshakeable resilience. For perspective, I will share circumstances and struggles that led me to the proverbial fork in the road. One road—the "easy" and "familiar"—would surely lead me to frustration and a life of continued misery. The other road—the "difficult" and "unfamiliar"—would potentially lead me to freedom and a life of peace and purpose.

Which did I choose? You can probably guess.

Do you enjoy traveling? I hope so because our story will take us on a journey in search of "The Recipe for Resilience." And what better way to discover "The Recipe for Resilience" than to journey to Resilience, USA. So, buckle up your seatbelt. You're exactly where you are supposed to be right now. This is your moment.

> *"We make our decisions, and then our decisions turn around and make us."*
>
> - F.W. Boreham

For as long as I can remember, I have preferred to be alone. As a young person, social situations brought me great anxiety. I never felt like I fit in anywhere. Friendships were very difficult for me to maintain.

You see, I was very overweight until about the age of 12. However, that insecure, "husky" young man disappeared between the summer of 7th and 8th grade. Practically overnight, it felt like I had brains, looks, and an appreciated athletic ability. Nevertheless, I was an incredibly insecure "popular" person. I didn't know how to handle it.

Then, one day, I made a decision that would have a profound impact on the rest of my life. I remember standing in the family kitchen. No one was home with me. I looked over to the corner of the dining room. There was a door with brown shutter-like slats pointing down. The solo, black handle called me to open the door like the Sirens calling out to Odysseus in Homer's Odyssey. I walked over and opened the door. I reached down for a bottle that looked familiar. A bottle that looked familiar from the many family parties that my parents hosted. I grabbed a glass. I slowly twisted off the cap. For some reason, I remember holding the bottle up to my nose and inhaling. The aroma was sweet. I inhaled deeply. Then, I poured. I drank. I was only 13 years old. I took my first alcoholic drink.

That decision led to one poor decision after another involving alcohol. As I entered high school, my "talent" for alcohol consumption continued to "improve." Alcohol didn't stop me from developing. It just prevented me from developing into the best version of myself. By the time I graduated from college with a BS in Accounting, I also graduated with an unofficial doctorate in alcohol abuse. Unfortunately, the alcohol abuse would continue for another 28 years.

A few years later, I was "reintroduced" to the love of my life. I met Patty when we were just children. Our families knew each other. She moved away when I was seven years old. Her grandmother would always say I was going to marry her. As fate would have it, we crossed paths again in our twenties after her grandfather died. I'll never, ever forget walking into her grandparent's house after arriving home from work on that cold December day on Hallock St. I was wearing my black winter overcoat. The coat and my slicked-back hair had me resembling someone from the movie "The Godfather." And there she was. Sitting in the corner was the most beautiful woman I had ever seen—wearing Kelly green sweatpants.

The courtship began long distance. I eventually moved to Florida, where we married. I brought myself—and my alcoholic self—into the marriage. Another person joined the marriage not long after—my verbally abusive self. This verbally abusive self increased as time went on. Altogether, I was a verbal abuser for 23 years of our 30-year relationship.

The alcohol abuse and verbal-abuser behavior fed into and created a vicious cycle of depression within me. Depression that would go dark and deep. Depression in which I wanted to take my life on multiple occasions. It's had a lasting impact on both my daughter and her mother. I am not proud to write about these things. However, I refuse to hide behind these masks anymore. I own what I have done 100 percent and accept the consequences of my decisions.

And then, in February 2016, my biggest fan and the person I most admired, my mother, died. This was a near fatal blow to me. I lost all confidence in myself, and I didn't think I had any more fight in me.

> *"If you're going through hell, keep going."*
>
> - Winston Churchill

Can a devil be redeemed? I have a lot of very smart people around me that I have added to my circle over the last few years. I can hear them now: "Don't call yourself a devil, Jim," or "Don't use those words to describe yourself, Jim." I get it. The fact of the matter is, however, that I did things that hurt other people—things that I knew were wrong. And now, the person I left my corporate career to care for was gone. I didn't know which direction to go without a career or caregiving. Even worse, I didn't trust myself or my decision-making.

There I was, standing at a fork in the road. Maybe you have stood at a fork in the road before. Maybe you are standing there right now. You must decide if you want to stay at a job you hate. You need to decide if you want to stay in a toxic relationship. You need to decide if you will continue to feed that addiction. Perhaps, you're facing a different fork in the road.

Whatever the fork, what is the common denominator? *You* must *decide* which way you want to go from here.

This is where our journey begins. I hope and pray that I can smooth out your life-learning curve by sharing the "Recipe for Resilience" that I discovered traveling along "The Road to Resilience."

I stood at the fork. I asked myself a question. Did I want to stay the man I was or was I going to work on becoming the man I truly wanted to be. I *decided*. I took my first step. I *decided* to step in the direction of becoming the man my wife and daughter would one day be proud of again.

If I stepped in this direction, I also *decided* that quitting was not an option. So, to increase the probability of my success, I knew that I would need to find the resilience to not give up. Throughout history, men and women have snatched success from the jaws of failure with one common trait: They simply refuse to accept failure. It was their resilience that brought them victory.

So, I simply *decided* that I wanted to change my life. I said goodbye to who I was and promised myself I would become who I was created to be.

I set the GPS for Resilience, USA. There were three stops to make along the journey, The Town of Foundation, Focusville, and the city known as Fundamental Formula. I hoped each stop would reveal something that would help me reach my goal of developing unwavering resilience.. So off I went.

> *"The important thing is that you've got a strong foundation before you start to try to save the world or help other people."*

> - Richard Branson

After a few hours of driving, I arrived at the town Foundation. I found a simple Airbnb on the edge of town with limited distractions. For the next few mornings, I kept to myself and took quiet walks in nature. I didn't interact much with the locals, but the weird thing is that all the people I did interact with seemed happy and at peace. I wondered what I was supposed to learn from this part of my journey. Finally, I decided to ask the owner of the Airbnb some questions, and I sensed that she'd been asked similar questions before. I also sensed that it was not a coincidence that I rented her place. I believe it was a divine appointment given to me as I stepped out in faith.

I will not soon forget what I learned there. The foundational principles exercised by the residents of Foundation had a great deal to do with their peace and happiness. I learned that they were people rooted in gratitude. They remain grateful in good times and bad, realizing there is always a lesson if you look close enough. Gratitude is the first foundational principle they build their lives on.

I'll never forget hearing the words from my host, "You can't control everything that happens to you, but you can control how you react to it Jim. ALWAYS, do your best to react in gratitude."

I also learned that the people of Foundation were early risers with a strong morning routine rooted in water intake, healthy nutrition, proper sleep, and continuous movement. These morning routines set the tone for their entire day.

As my stop at Foundation ended, I made sure to express proper gratitude to my host for the valuable foundational information I learned and vowed to apply it to my life. Her final words were probably the most important: "Resilience requires a strong *foundation* applied *consistently*."

*"Don't look at the wall. Your car goes where your eyes go."*

- Mario Andretti

I was looking forward to my next stop. It would be an overnight visit with an old friend who moved to a small town named Focusville to simplify his life.

We agreed to meet at a local coffee shop. My buddy said that the place had the best and freshest desserts, all handmade from scratch. He mentioned that the pumpkin cheesecake was to die for, and he knew I was a sucker for a good pumpkin cheesecake. "A small indulgence every now and then is OK," he reminded me.

Our visit was just like old times. We caught up on everything. What got my attention the most was just how present my buddy was. In fact, unlike most people I visit with, his cell phone was nowhere to be found. When I brought this up to my friend, he proceeded to teach me a valuable lesson.

The more my friend talked about where the real power lies today, I realized he was revealing something valuable. He said, "Real power lies in those who can focus. Information does not have the same power like it used to. Need to know something? Just Google it! But today's overly distracted and overly stimulated lives require intense *focus*." This realization alone showed me how distracted I had allowed myself to be in the past. And those distractions quite often lead to me making poor choices.

I left Focusville with a firm understanding that where my eyes and ears go, my life will follow. If I was going to lead a life of peace and purpose, it would require me to guard my eyes and ears. I would consistently flush out negativity with positive, life-giving thoughts and energy. In doing this, I would increase the probability of being successful in developing resilience.

*"Simple can be harder than complex: You have to work hard to get your thinking clean to make it simple. But it's worth it in the end because once you get there, you can move mountains."*

- Steve Jobs

My final stop on the road to resilience landed me in the city I would come to know as the great city of Fundamental Formula. I wondered what I needed to learn from this stop on the journey. I became more energized and hopeful as I reflected on what I had learned about building a strong *foundation* and applying intense *focus*.

I began to *intentionally look inward*. I removed the masks I had been hiding behind for many years. I felt reborn, living a more authentic life. The personal development I was applying was certainly helping me grow into the man I was created to be.

However, a shift was occurring. It was here I realized that it wasn't even about me anymore. So, I committed to humble myself and *intentionally look outward and upward* by adding spiritual development to my personal development. I knew there was something bigger than me—something I could ask for help. Together, the personal and spiritual development created a power that gave me hope I hadn't felt in a very long time.

However, my work was taking me longer than I thought it would. This issue revealed a third piece of development to me. In fact, it would turn out to be the secret sauce in "The Recipe for Resilience." There is immense power in this form of development. I call it the power of intentional connecting or relational development.

Personal development looks inward. Spiritual development looks out and up. Relational development looks intentionally into the hearts of others. Once we look into their hearts, we try to add value to their lives. Sometimes, we connect with people who we want to add to our circle. Other times, we learn that we need to prune them from our lives. Ultimately, relational development is about having the people in your life that value who you are and value who you are becoming. I realized *this* was the *formula* I needed to apply once I built a strong *foundation* and developed intense *focus*.

And just like that, a wave of peace and purpose overcame me to tears. The "Recipe for Resilience" was revealed:

Foundation + Focus + Formula = Freedom

I began to wonder. Was it really this simple? Then I remembered the Steve Jobs quote above. Simple can move mountains. Simple can develop resilience. Resilience will help you overcome anything. The "Road to Resilience" is not a place you need to go. It already resides inside you. It's your job to find it. Do the work. I promise you that it's worth it.

*"Love, Love, Love. All you need is love. Love is all you need."*

- John Lennon

I hope this story provided some nuggets to help you along your journey. I am grateful for the opportunity to share things that you might use to improve your life and overcome obstacles that may be holding you back from living the life you were created to live.

Always remember, at the end of it all, we're not here for very long. So, forgive yourself and others. Never stop learning how to love yourself and love others. It's the best gift you can give yourself and the world.

Develop the resilience to overcome any obstacle. And don't ever be afraid to *pivot with purpose*!

# Harnessing the Power of Positive Thinking: Minimizing Anxiety through Eliminating Negative Self-Talk

BY
LISA A. JONES

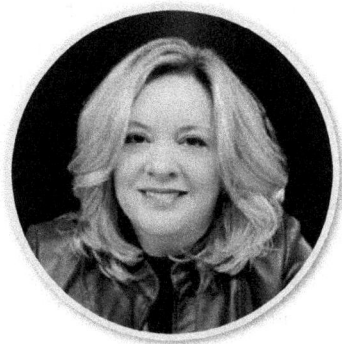

Residing in the bustling metropolis of Minneapolis, Lisa, an accomplished resume writer and philanthropist, leads a life filled with exciting activities. As the CEO of a nonprofit organization dedicated to assisting individuals worldwide, she appeared to be content and fulfilled. However, beneath her confident exterior lay a hidden battle: the constant onslaught of negative self-talk.

Every day, while engrossed in various projects, Lisa found herself engaged in an internal dialogue. She would meticulously analyze her every action, questioning her abilities and doubting her value. This never-ending stream of self-criticism gradually eroded her confidence and diminished her overall happiness.

One ordinary day at work, as she sat at her desk pondering over a new assignment with furrowed brows, Lisa stumbled upon an article discussing negative self-talk. Curiosity piqued within her as she delved into this concept to gain insight into her struggles. Much to her astonishment and relief, she discovered that countless others experienced similar challenges along their journey toward self-acceptance.

***That Lisa, is me.***

The phenomenon of negative self-talk impacts many individuals without their conscious awareness. This incessant internal dialogue, characterized by self-criticism, doubt, and pessimism, can profoundly affect mental well-being. The words we utter to ourselves hold significance; thus, negative self-talk contributes to feelings of anxiety, diminished self-worth, and even depression. Recognizing the correlation between negative self-talk and anxiety is crucial to effectively mitigate its influence. I experienced this firsthand when my sense of esteem plummeted to such an extent that I would cancel meetings out of fear—fear that I might say something foolish—ultimately causing me to forfeit meaningful opportunities.

Many of us wonder what we did to make someone else act rudely to us, playing this back over in our minds trying to find an answer. As we do this, our anxiety worsens because there isn't an answer most of the time. Anxiety can be overwhelming and debilitating, affecting many aspects of our lives. We commonly find ourselves caught in a loop of self-doubt and self-blame, pondering, *"Why? Why? Why?"*

No matter how much we analyze situations, the behavior of others ultimately lies within their emotions and choices. While it can be frustrating and disheartening, it is essential for our well-being to recognize we cannot fix or change the way others treat us. Instead of dwelling on the actions of others, we have the power to shift our focus toward self-care.

We must prioritize our mental and emotional well-being by distancing ourselves from toxic relationships. By choosing to walk away from negativity, we create space for positive experiences and healthier interactions. Remember, many factors can trigger anxiety, and one of them is placing too much importance on the actions and opinions of others.

When it comes to combating anxiety, one effective strategy is to replace negative thoughts with positive ones. I know this isn't always easy, but it's necessary. Negative thoughts have a way of creeping back in when we least expect them. But, with a little practice, we can shift our mindset toward a more positive light.

Try recalling moments that brought you happiness. Reflect on instances where you achieved something significant, like receiving a good grade on a paper or playing your best round of golf. These accomplishments serve as reminders of your capabilities and can help boost your self-esteem. Replaying compliments in your mind can have a profound impact. Think back to a time when someone genuinely praised you, making you smile and raise your head with pride. Revisit that moment and let those positive feelings surround you.

Remembering acts of kindness and moments when you brought joy to someone's life can also help with anxiety. These memories can be a powerful tool to combat negative thoughts and promote a positive outlook. We can gradually replace negative thoughts by consciously redirecting our thoughts toward positive experiences. It may take time and practice, but with dedication, we can cultivate a more optimistic mindset.

Tackling anxiety is an ongoing process, and it is essential to be patient with yourself. Embrace the journey of self-improvement and celebrate the smallest victories along the way. We cultivate a sense of inner peace and resilience by redirecting our energy toward self-reflection and personal growth. So, let go of the need for answers that may never come and embrace the power you have to create a better life for yourself.

## THE CONNECTION BETWEEN NEGATIVE SELF-TALK AND ANXIETY

The connection between negative self-talk and anxiety is deeply intertwined, as they tend to feed off each other in a destructive loop. Engaging in negative self-talk reinforces and amplifies our worries, ultimately leading to heightened anxiety levels. Our thoughts profoundly impact our emotions, so constantly subjecting ourselves to self-criticism only intensifies stress responses and triggers anxious thoughts. For instance, repeatedly convincing ourselves that we are inadequate or bound to fail cultivates a pervasive feeling of apprehension and unease. Recognizing this intricate relationship is pivotal in breaking free from the cycle and alleviating anxiety.

## EXAMPLES OF NEGATIVE SELF-TALK AND ITS EFFECTS ON MENTAL WELL-BEING

Negative self-talk can manifest in various ways, and its effects can harm mental well-being.

Common examples include:

1.  **Personalization**: Blaming oneself for circumstances beyond our control can result in feelings of guilt and diminished self-worth. This mindset involves constantly assuming responsibility for events or outcomes that lie outside one's sphere of influence. For instance, if a friend cancels plans due to a family emergency, an individual who internalizes may think, *It's my fault; they don't want to be around me,* even though the friend's situation has no connection to them whatsoever. Such self-blame perpetuates negative emotions and hampers one's ability to recognize external factors at play.

2.  **Catastrophizing**: Catastrophizing is a cognitive distortion characterized by the tendency to amplify and exaggerate the potential negative consequence of a situation. This thought pattern involves envisioning the worst possible outcome and believing it is highly probable, even without substantial evidence supporting such beliefs. Individuals engaging in this thought process often blow minor setbacks or inconveniences out of proportion. This can lead to excessive worry, anxiety, and stress. It can influence behavior by causing individuals to avoid certain situations or take extreme measures to prevent the imagined catastrophe.

    For instance, let's consider someone anticipating a performance review at work. If they indulge in catastrophizing thoughts, they might think, *I am certain I will receive an awful review. My boss will criticize all my work, and I will most likely be terminated.* In reality, there may be no concrete evidence supporting such a disastrous outcome; however, this person's thoughts are fixated on the worst-case scenario.

Catastrophizing can have detrimental effects on one's mental well-being as well as decision-making abilities. It is crucial for individuals to acknowledge this thinking pattern and challenge its validity through rational analysis of facts rather than succumbing to irrational fears based solely on imagination or speculation.

3. **Overgeneralization**: Overgeneralization is a cognitive distortion where individuals draw broad and negative conclusions about themselves, others, or the world based on isolated incidents or limited experiences. In this type of thinking, a single negative event is seen as evidence that everything will always be negative.

   For example, if someone goes on a date that doesn't go well and they think, *I'm terrible at relationships. I'll never find love*, they are overgeneralizing based on one isolated incident. In reality, one bad date does not predict the outcome of future relationships.

   Overgeneralization can also affect how individuals perceive and interact with others, leading them to make unfair assumptions about people or situations. Looking for evidence to support or contradict the negative conclusion can help gain a more balanced perspective.

4. **Labeling**: Labeling is a cognitive distortion where individuals assign derogatory labels to themselves based on perceived shortcomings or mistakes. It involves making global, sweeping judgments about one's character or identity based on specific behaviors or situations. This type of thinking can be extremely damaging to self-esteem and self-image. For example, if someone makes a mistake at work, they might label themselves "stupid" or "a failure." We must remember that making a mistake is a normal part of being human and does not define our entire worth or intelligence.

To combat labeling, practicing self-compassion and challenging negative self-judgments is essential. Recognizing that making mistakes is a natural part of life and does not diminish one's overall value. Engaging in positive self-talk and acknowledging one's strengths and accomplishments can counteract the negative impact of labeling.

In a world of diverse opinions, it is impossible to please everyone. Trying to do so will only increase our anxiety levels. Therefore, it is important to remember that showing ourselves compassion and kindness is acceptable and necessary.

5. **Should statements**: In the realm of self-criticism, sometimes we impose unrealistic expectations upon ourselves or others and subsequently criticize ourselves when these expectations are not met. Such thinking frequently involves the use of words like "should," "must," "ought to," or "have to" in reference to how things ought to be or how one should conduct themselves. We all experience those moments when we reflect on what we should have done, could have done, or would have done differently.

For example, if someone is struggling to complete a task, they might think, *I should be able to do this easily. I'm such a failure for not being able to handle it.* The individual sets an unrealistic expectation that the task should be effortless for them, and when it proves challenging, they criticize themselves. Should statements can lead to feelings of inadequacy and frustration. They can also contribute to a negative cycle of self-blame and self-criticism. We may never feel satisfied with our accomplishments by holding onto these unrealistic expectations, even when we are doing our best.

To address should statements, it's essential to recognize when they occur and challenge their validity. Embracing a more flexible and compassionate attitude toward oneself, where it's okay to have limitations and make mistakes, can lead to a healthier and more balanced perspective.

***Dismiss those intrusive thoughts of "should've, would've, could've" when they arise and banish them from your mind.***

## COGNITIVE BEHAVIORAL THERAPY (CBT) AND ITS ROLE IN CHALLENGING NEGATIVE THOUGHTS

At times, it is necessary to seek assistance from a skilled professional. It is important to remember that we cannot accomplish everything on our own and that reaching out for help demonstrates strength.

CBT, also referred to as cognitive behavioral therapy, is a widely recognized and effective form of psychotherapy. This versatile approach can be applied to treat various mental health concerns and address emotional and behavioral difficulties.

The principles that underpin cognitive behavioral therapy have been outlined by the American Psychological Association (APA). According to these principles:

1.  Psychological issues often stem from distorted or unproductive thought patterns.
2.  Maladaptive behaviors learned over time contribute to psychological problems.
3.  Individuals experiencing psychological challenges can learn healthier coping mechanisms, ultimately alleviating their symptoms and enhancing their overall functioning.

By adhering to these core principles, cognitive behavioral therapy provides individuals with the tools they need to challenge negative thinking patterns, modify harmful behaviors, and develop more adaptive strategies for managing their emotions and circumstances. Through this process of growth and change, individuals can achieve improved mental well-being and lead more fulfilling lives (Radias Health, 2023).

CBT focuses on identifying and challenging distorted thoughts and replacing them with more realistic and positive alternatives. By understanding the connection between our thoughts, emotions, and behaviors, CBT empowers individuals to break free from negative thinking patterns.

Individuals learn to identify negative self-talk and question its validity. They are encouraged to examine the evidence for and against their negative thoughts, challenging their assumptions and biases. By doing so, they can replace negative self-talk with more balanced and realistic thoughts, leading to reduced anxiety and improved mental well-being. CBT exercises for anxiety often involve keeping thought records, analyzing cognitive distortions, and developing coping strategies.

## PRACTICAL EXERCISES TO REPLACE NEGATIVE SELF-TALK

Challenging and replacing negative self-talk requires practice and perseverance. Below are some practical exercises to help you get started:

**Identify and analyze**: Start by becoming aware of your negative self-talk patterns. Write down any negative thoughts you notice and analyze them objectively. Are they based on facts or distorted perceptions?

**Question the evidence**: Challenge the validity of your negative thoughts. Ask yourself if there is concrete evidence to support them. Are you jumping to conclusions without considering alternative explanations?

**Replace with positive affirmations**: Develop a list of positive affirmations that counteract your negative self-talk. Repeat them regularly to rewire your thought patterns and cultivate a more positive mindset.

**Practice self-compassion**: Treat yourself with kindness and understanding. Replace self-criticism with self-compassion, acknowledging that everyone makes mistakes and that you deserve love and acceptance.

## THE POWER OF POSITIVE AFFIRMATIONS

Positive affirmations are powerful tools for cultivating a confident mindset. Individuals can rewire their thought patterns and boost self-confidence by intentionally repeating positive statements about themselves. Positive affirmations help challenge and replace negative thoughts, promoting a more optimistic and empowering internal dialogue. Incorporate positive affirmations into your daily routine and witness the transformative impact on your mental well-being.

An effective practice that I have discovered is to develop a habit of consciously reflecting on the positive aspects of each day. By taking a few moments to write down something positive that occurred and expressing gratitude for it, I have experienced a profound shift in my mindset. I created a jar dedicated to collecting these joyful memories to keep track of these moments. Adding these notes to the jar at the end of each day has become a wonderful ritual.

As the days turn into weeks and months, this jar of positivity serves as a powerful reminder of the goodness in my life. When I take the time to read through these notes at the end of each month, I am filled with an even deeper sense of appreciation and gratitude. It's truly amazing how these moments, which might have otherwise been forgotten, continue to bring a smile to my face and a warm feeling to my heart.

On the other hand, I have also implemented a similar practice for dealing with negative thoughts. Whenever I find myself repeatedly dwelling on something negative, I have developed the habit of jotting it down on a piece of paper and placing it in a separate jar. This act of acknowledging and releasing these negative thoughts has proven remarkably therapeutic for me. At the end of each week, I safely burn these to never be read again.

In doing so, I intentionally let go of these negative feelings and made room for more positive energy and mindset. This simple yet powerful act has helped me avoid getting trapped in a cycle of negativity. It has allowed me to focus on cultivating a more optimistic and uplifting outlook on life.

These self-healing positive practices of collecting affirmative moments and releasing negative thoughts in separate jars have significantly enhanced my entire life. By consciously choosing to focus on the positive and letting go of the negative, I have experienced a transformation in my mindset and outlook.

*I encourage you all to try this practice, as it can bring about meaningful changes in one's life.*

## INCORPORATING MINDFULNESS AND SELF-COMPASSION

Mindfulness and self-compassion are complementary practices that can effectively combat negative self-talk and reduce anxiety. Mindfulness involves being fully present in the moment, observing thoughts and emotions without judgment. By cultivating mindfulness, individuals can develop a greater awareness of their negative self-talk and choose not to engage with it. Self-compassion, on the other hand, involves treating oneself with kindness and understanding, especially in moments of struggle. By practicing self-compassion, individuals can counteract self-criticism and foster a more supportive and nurturing inner voice.

*I understand that I've mentioned this before, but it cannot be stressed enough how important it is to practice self-compassion.*

## The Importance of Seeking Professional Help for Severe Anxiety and Negative Self-Talk

While self-help strategies can be effective for many individuals, it is essential to recognize when professional help is necessary. Severe anxiety and persistent negative self-talk may require the guidance of a mental health professional. Therapists trained in CBT can provide personalized strategies and support in managing anxiety. Seeking professional help is a sign of strength and a proactive step toward improving mental well-being.

## Conclusion

Harnessing the power of positive thinking and minimizing anxiety through eliminating negative self-talk is a transformative journey that requires commitment and self-reflection. You can break free from the cycle of negativity by understanding the connection, challenging distorted thoughts, and incorporating positive affirmations, mindfulness, and self-compassion.

Embrace the power of positive thinking and witness its profound impact on your mental well-being.

I hope that as you go through the pages of this book, you find some healing tips that resonate with you. It is said that we all have our battles to fight, but what is truly remarkable is how we can come together and help one another along the way. This book was crafted with the intention of providing guidance and support to those who may be seeking it. Whether it's through sharing personal experiences, offering practical advice, or simply providing a comforting voice, this book aims to extend a helping hand to anyone who may need it. So, remember, let's continue to be there for each other, offering support and kindness as we navigate life's challenges. Because together, we can make a difference.

***Namaste***

## REFERENCES

Radias Health. (2023, February 23). *What is cognitive behavioral therapy?* https://radiashealth.org/what-is-cognitive-behavioral-therapy/?gclid=CjwKCAjwlJimBhAs EiwA1hrp5mDtTO-F-7DtrNw0Y-0OGwyEnWGik F_IKmpiGbeOIpyUFKJZOWGLyBoCYroQAvD_BwE

# How the Mind Manages Money: Navigating Financial Challenges in Good and Bad Times

## By
## Rick Loek

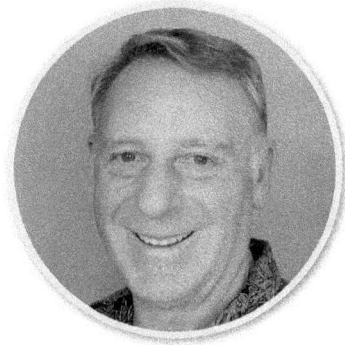

Certain life events are permanently etched into your mind—the birth of a child, the death of a parent, the deaths of key people in your life, and so on. The COVID-19 Pandemic is one of those life events.

❄ For those who like a softer introduction to this subject, consider reading the paragraphs that start with an ❄. These are hypothetical stories and share the same concept via a story.

Let me take you back to the Big Island of Hawaii, where my wife and I were immersed in a transformative Huna training. Surrounded by over 200 individuals seeking ancient Hawaiian healing and energy arts, it was a powerful and enlightening experience. Meanwhile, amid this paradise, my mind was still occupied by the responsibilities of running my investment advisor company.

Being responsible for managing my clients' assets, I implemented a program designed to protect their investments in case of a catastrophic event. This program would automatically shift their assets to cash, safeguarding their wealth. It seemed like a stroke of luck that such a safety net existed during uncertain times.

Or so I thought.

As the stock market experienced a period of unprecedented volatility, I anticipated that all my clients' investments would be converted to cash, adhering to the program's design. However, to my surprise, I discovered another option available to my clients—a "downgrade" of their asset mix. This alternative required accurate manual input from humans into the computer system, a step I was unaware of at the time.

When I logged in to check, I discovered that many of my clients' accounts were still fully invested, albeit with a "downgraded" status. Perplexed and concerned, I immediately contacted the back-office team to seek clarification. They assured me that these clients had indeed chosen the "downgrade" option as part of their investment strategy.

Here I was, amidst the breathtaking beauty of Hawaii, while my clients' accounts and the world faced financial catastrophe. I couldn't ignore the situation. Determined to rectify this oversight, I found myself burning the midnight oil, meticulously auditing each client account. I needed concrete evidence to support my claim that these clients had not intentionally chosen the "downgrade" option. Apart from one client and one account, it became evident that my intuition was correct.

For the following months, I tirelessly worked with the back-office team, urging them to rectify their mistakes and make my clients whole again. Making them whole meant the company took responsibility for their errors and retroactively executed trades to correct the financial discrepancies. The gravity of the situation was staggering, with some clients facing losses exceeding $100,000.

Finally, after the last client had been compensated, I decided to sever ties with that back-office team. Their lack of attention to detail and the magnitude of their errors left me with no choice but to seek a more reliable partner. It was a bittersweet moment, knowing that my clients were made whole, but also realizing the need to rebuild their trust in a new partnership.

Despite the challenges faced in that paradise setting, the experience served as a stark reminder of the importance of diligence and oversight when entrusted with managing others' financial well-being. It reinforced my commitment to providing my clients with the utmost care and attention, ensuring that their investments are safeguarded, and their trust is unwavering.

Today, let's embark on a fascinating journey exploring how our minds handle the delicate dance of managing money. Money impacts our choices, security, and overall well-being, and understanding the psychological and emotional aspects of financial management is crucial. In this chapter, we'll delve into the different scenarios of having too much or not enough money, navigating both good and bad times. We'll also explore the mental and emotional challenges people faced at the start of the pandemic. Finally, we'll provide you with five strategies for overcoming any money-related issues that come your way. Get ready to dive into the intriguing world of the mind and money.

**NOTE:** ❁ Below are fictional scenarios highlighting the stress experienced by individuals with different financial circumstances. The purpose is to emphasize the psychological and emotional challenges faced by both those with too much and too little money.

I.   **Having Too Much Money:** Having abundant wealth can be both a dream come true and a challenge in disguise. Let's explore how the mind handles having too much money and the complexities it can bring.

Guilt and Responsibility: When sudden wealth enters our lives, it's common to experience guilt or question whether we truly deserve such abundance. The mind may wrestle with feelings of responsibility and the urge to positively impact the world.

❁Meet Amelia, a successful tech entrepreneur who catapulted into immense wealth overnight after her company went public. While grateful for her financial success, Amelia couldn't shake the overwhelming guilt accompanying her newfound riches. She questioned whether she deserved such abundance when countless others struggled to make ends meet. Determined to alleviate her guilt, Amelia embarked on a journey to positively impact the world. She established charitable foundations, supported causes close to her heart, and dedicated herself to philanthropy, using her wealth as a force for good.

Fear and Insecurity: Surprisingly, even with vast riches, fear and insecurity can creep into our minds. The fear of losing our wealth or the insecurity of maintaining our status can cloud our decision-making, making us more cautious and less willing to take calculated risks.

❊Enter Sebastian, an heir to a vast family fortune who always had the best that money could buy. Despite his opulent lifestyle, Sebastian found himself haunted by fear and insecurity. The weight of preserving his family's legacy and the constant pressure to maintain his status in high society burdened his mind. Fearful of losing his wealth and the accompanying privileges, Sebastian became risk-averse, often missing out on potential opportunities. Through self-reflection and seeking professional guidance, he gradually learned to manage his fear and insecurity, embracing calculated risks and finding a healthier balance between caution and growth.

**Loss of Purpose and Identity:** Excessive wealth can sometimes blur our sense of purpose and identity. Without financial struggles, we may grapple with questions like, "Who am I beyond my wealth?" The mind seeks a deeper understanding of self-worth and fulfillment beyond material achievements.

❊In this story, we meet Olivia, a self-made millionaire who started a successful fashion empire. As her wealth multiplied, Olivia felt disconnected from her true passions and questioned her identity beyond material achievements. The allure of luxury and financial success began to overshadow her sense of purpose. Olivia embarked on a soul-searching journey, seeking clarity and exploring different avenues to reconnect with her authentic self. She pursued her long-lost hobbies, engaged in meaningful volunteer work, and discovered a passion for mentoring aspiring entrepreneurs. Through this process, Olivia redefined her purpose, finding fulfillment in inspiring others and embracing a more balanced and purpose-driven life.

II. **Not Having Enough Money:** On the flip side, not having enough money can bring about stress, anxiety, and constant financial struggles. Let's explore how the mind copes with financial scarcity and the challenges it presents.

**Stress and Anxiety:** Financial scarcity can cause chronic stress and anxiety as we worry about making ends meet and managing debts. The mind becomes preoccupied with survival, hindering our ability to think long-term or focus on other important aspects of life.

❋Meet Ethan, a hardworking individual who, despite his best efforts, constantly finds himself struggling to make ends meet. The weight of financial scarcity bears down on him, leading to chronic stress and anxiety. Every bill, every unexpected expense becomes a source of worry and preoccupation. Constantly juggling limited resources leaves little mental space for long-term planning or pursuing other important aspects of life. To cope with this stress, Ethan seeks support from counseling services and engages in mindfulness practices to regain a sense of calm and find resilience amidst the financial challenges.

**Limited Choices and Opportunities:** A lack of financial resources limits our choices and opportunities. Education, career advancement, and even leisure activities may seem out of reach. The mind becomes fixated on finding immediate solutions, leaving little room for long-term planning or pursuing our passions.

❋Enter Maya, a talented young artist with a passion for painting. Unfortunately, her financial circumstances limit her choices and opportunities. Unable to afford higher education or art supplies, Maya feels trapped in a cycle of limited options. The mind becomes fixated on immediate survival, leaving little room for pursuing her artistic passion. However, Maya refuses to let her circumstances define her. She seeks out local art communities, connects with mentors, and discovers online platforms to showcase and sell her artwork. Through resilience and resourcefulness, she finds creative ways to pursue her passion and open new opportunities.

**Social Stigma and Shame:** In societies that place significant importance on financial success, insufficient money can lead to shame and embarrassment. The mind may struggle with feelings of inadequacy and isolation, further compounding the emotional burden.

❋In this story, we meet Daniel, a dedicated individual who faces financial scarcity and its social stigma. Living in a society that places significant emphasis on material success, Daniel experiences feelings of shame and inadequacy due to his financial struggles. He fears being judged by others and feels isolated from social circles that revolve around affluence. However, Daniel realizes that his self-worth extends beyond his financial situation. He seeks support from support groups and engages in self-empowerment activities that boost his confidence and help him overcome the social stigma. Eventually, Daniel finds solace in building genuine connections with others based on shared values and experiences rather than financial status.

**III. The Mental and Emotional Challenges of the Pandemic:** The COVID-19 pandemic brought unprecedented challenges, shaking economies and causing financial turmoil globally. Let's explore people's mental and emotional hurdles during these uncertain times.

**Fear and Uncertainty:** The pandemic unleashed a wave of fear and uncertainty, affecting our financial decision-making. With the fear of contracting the virus and the economic instability, the mind found itself caught in a web of anxiety, making it difficult to think clearly.

❋Meet Sarah, a young professional accustomed to a stable job and financial security. However, when the pandemic hit, fear and uncertainty took hold of her mind. She worried about the risk of contracting the virus and the economic instability it brought. The fear paralyzed her decision-making, making it difficult to think clearly about her finances. Sarah sought support from online communities and counseling services to cope with this challenge. Through sharing her fears and receiving guidance, she gradually learned to manage her anxiety and make more rational financial decisions amidst the uncertainty.

**Emotional Rollercoaster:** As financial markets fluctuated and incomes dwindled, our emotions went on a wild ride. Frustration, despair, and a sense of helplessness became constant companions as we grappled with the rapidly changing circumstances.

❋In this story, we meet Alex, a business owner who experienced an emotional rollercoaster during the pandemic. As the financial markets fluctuated and his income dwindled, he found himself on a constant emotional rollercoaster ride. Frustration, despair, and a sense of helplessness became his constant companions. To navigate this challenging emotional terrain, Alex engaged in regular journaling and sought support from loved ones. He learned to recognize and acknowledge his emotions without allowing them to control his decision-making. With time, he developed resilience and the ability to find moments of calm amidst the storm.

**Increased Financial Pressure:** The pandemic intensified financial pressure, leading to worries about meeting basic needs, paying bills, and maintaining our desired lifestyle. The mind felt overwhelmed, contributing to heightened anxiety, depression, and other mental health issues.

❋Enter Rachel, a single parent facing increased financial pressure due to the pandemic. With job losses, reduced hours, and the rising cost of living, Rachel's worries about meeting basic needs and paying bills intensified. The mind felt overwhelmed, leading to heightened anxiety, depression, and other mental health issues. Rachel contacted local community resources, such as food banks and financial assistance programs, to help alleviate the immediate financial pressure. She also engaged in therapy to address the underlying mental health challenges. Through these resources and support, Rachel gradually regained control and stability in her financial and emotional well-being.

IV. **Five Strategies for Overcoming Money-Related Issues:** Now that we've explored the mind's journey through different financial scenarios, let's equip ourselves with five powerful strategies to overcome money-related challenges.

**Mindful Budgeting:** Develop a comprehensive budget that aligns with your financial goals and values. Approach spending mindfully, ensuring your choices reflect your priorities and bring you closer to your desired financial state.

❋Meet Kristine, a young professional struggling with mounting debt and a lack of financial clarity. Determined to regain control of her finances, she embarked on a journey of mindful budgeting. Kristine meticulously analyzed her income, expenses, and financial goals, creating a comprehensive budget aligned with her values. With each purchasing decision, she asked herself if it brought her closer to her desired financial state. By approaching spending mindfully and making conscious choices, Kristine managed to pay off her debts and started saving toward her long-term goals.

**Cultivate a Growth Mindset:** Embrace a growth mindset regarding money. See setbacks as opportunities for growth and improvement. Stay open to learning new financial strategies and exploring avenues for income generation.

❋Enter Juan, an aspiring entrepreneur who faced several setbacks and financial challenges along the way. Rather than letting these setbacks discourage him, Juan embraced a growth mindset regarding money. He saw each setback as an opportunity for growth and improvement. He sought financial education resources, attended workshops, and learned from successful entrepreneurs. With a willingness to adapt and learn, Juan eventually turned his financial situation around, leveraging new strategies and income-generating avenues to achieve success.

**Seek Professional Guidance:** Consult with financial advisors or experts who can provide objective guidance tailored to your circumstances. Their expertise can help you make informed decisions and alleviate financial stress.

❋In this story, we meet James, a middle-aged individual who felt overwhelmed by the complexity of his financial decisions. Unsure of how to navigate his financial challenges, James decided to seek professional guidance. He consulted with a financial advisor who provided objective advice tailored to his specific circumstances. With the guidance and expertise of the financial advisor, James gained clarity and confidence in making informed financial decisions. This guidance alleviated his financial stress and set him on a path toward achieving his long-term financial goals.

**Build Financial Resilience:** Prioritize building a financial safety net by setting aside an emergency fund. This buffer can provide peace of mind and mitigate the stress associated with financial uncertainties.

❋Enter Ellen, a young professional who recognized the importance of building a financial safety net. Despite her limited income, Ellen prioritized setting aside a portion of her earnings into an emergency fund. Over time, this fund grew, providing her with a sense of security and peace of mind. When unexpected expenses or financial uncertainties arose, Ellen had a buffer to rely on, reducing the stress associated with financial emergencies. This financial resilience empowered her to face challenges confidently and maintain stability in her financial life.

**Prioritize Self-Care:** Invest in your mental and emotional well-being. Engage in activities that reduce stress, such as exercise, meditation, or pursuing hobbies. Positively nurturing your overall well-being impacts your financial decision-making.

❀In this story, we meet Michael, a working parent who experienced constant stress and anxiety due to financial pressures. Recognizing the toll it was taking on his mental and emotional well-being, Michael prioritized self-care as a strategy for overcoming money-related issues. He invested time in activities that reduced stress, such as regular exercise, meditation, and pursuing his hobbies. By nurturing his overall well-being, Michael made better financial decisions and approached money matters with a clearer mindset. This self-care practice contributed to his overall financial well-being and improved his quality of life.

As we wrap up this exploration of how the mind manages money, remember that financial management goes beyond numbers. By understanding the psychological and emotional aspects, we can navigate the complexities of having too much or not enough money. The challenges faced during the pandemic further highlighted the importance of a resilient mindset. By implementing strategies like mindful budgeting, cultivating a growth mindset, seeking professional guidance, building financial resilience, and prioritizing self-care, we can overcome money-related issues and create a healthier relationship with our finances. Your mind is a powerful tool, capable of managing money with wisdom and grace. Embrace the journey, and may your financial path be paved with abundance and prosperity!

I am developing a curriculum centered around money, focusing on helping individuals like you transform your relationship with finances and remove the hidden constraints that prevent you from living life to the fullest.

I am an enthusiast for personal connection and community. I invite you to reach out via email or phone for mentoring, coaching, focus sessions, or breakthrough sessions. All of my contact information is located and kept current at http://TheAmazingRick.com

# Unlocking the Power Within: Transforming Anxiety into Empowerment with 3 Simple Tools

### BY
### Ronita Godsi

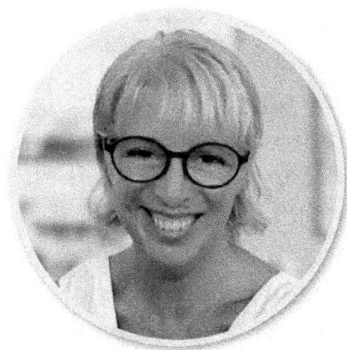

You know that feeling when you're stuck and keep asking yourself, "What should I do?" It's like being torn between two options: to love or to leave, to quit or to stay, to do it or not, to buy it or not, to say it or keep it inside. The problem is, when you're so close to the issue, it's hard to see any solutions, let alone the opportunities that might exist.

Deep down, we all instinctively know that life will remain difficult if we stay stuck in the same mental state. It's not living; at best, it's merely existing. If you're ready to break free from this cycle, let me share the three tools I used to create just a two-millimeter shift in my focus and, consequently, my life.

But before I dive into that, let me tell you a bit about my story. I want to share how I overcame months of overwhelm, panic, and freezing in the face of debilitating fear.

I still remember that night when everything seemed to crumble around me. It was two o'clock in the morning in Los Angeles—too early to disturb my Mum in London and too late to reach out to my sister in LA. Overwhelmed by the weight of my pain, I longed to just make that pain stop. It felt easier to check out of life.

Sitting there, feeling lost and uncertain, I found myself inexplicably drawn to my laptop. A voice echoed in my mind, urging me to pick it up and do something, anything. Through what felt like divine intervention, I discovered Tony Robbins and his program, "The Ultimate Edge." It offered a lifeline—a 30-day trial that allowed me to return it within the same timeframe, avoiding the hefty $997 price tag. With only $34 left in my dwindling bank account and $30 for shipping, I stood at a crossroads. In that agonizing space of decision, survival mode kicked in, and I experienced a deep knowing within me that this was the path I needed to take. So, I invested that $30 into Tony Robbins' program—an investment in myself.

In that fragile moment, I struck a deal with higher powers. "Just get me through to daylight," I pleaded, promising to pay it forward when the time came. As I made that payment, I felt immense gratitude when I discovered that Tony Robbins provided two hours of audio material I could instantly download. I clung to those recordings as if my life depended on them because it did. Throughout the night, they played on an endless loop, replacing the tormenting voice in my head with one of strength, resilience, and hope.

Hour by hour, I endured, inching closer to the break of day. That night marked a rock bottom, a point that threatened to consume me entirely. But even in the depths of despair, I couldn't ignore my sense of responsibility. I couldn't leave my four precious daughters, whose souls had been entrusted to me, in the hands of someone who had inflicted such pain—especially now that I understood the full extent of his actions. I believed I had no choice but to carry on.

So, I made a deal with myself. All I would require of myself was making a mere two millimeters of progress daily. Some days, that meant staying in bed, summoning the strength to rise only for my daughters—to take them to school, pick them up, and provide them with dinner—before retreating to the safety of my covers. It was a journey of survival, juggling four or sometimes five jobs at a time, tirelessly striving for any future different from this agony.

Panic attacks would grip me whenever his number appeared on my phone screen. Yet, in those moments of paralyzing fear, I found solace in the audios—Tony Robbins' unwavering voice and Esther Hicks' uplifting wisdom. I played them on a loop, allowing their words to fill my being, instilling within me a dominant intent to see the positive or at least anything different from what I was currently experiencing.

Slowly, ever so slowly, I began to emerge from the suffocating abyss that had engulfed me. Each step forward, no matter how small, carried profound significance. With resilience as my guide, I navigated the labyrinth of darkness, finding moments of light along the way.

## RELIEF:

These simple yet incredibly powerful tools became my lifeline, guiding me through the tumultuous journey of life, moment by moment. They were the keys that unlocked my ability to navigate overwhelming waves of panic and paralyzing fear.

These tools were not elaborate or complex, but their impact was immeasurable. They allowed me to reclaim my power and rise above the suffocating grip of fear and anxiety. Through their simplicity, I discovered the profound truth that sometimes the most effective tools are the ones that speak directly to our hearts and souls.

Day by day, minute by minute, they propelled me forward, enabling me to transcend the barriers that once held me captive. These simple yet transformative tools have forever changed the way I navigate life's challenges. They are a constant reminder of my inner power and the limitless possibilities within me. With their help, I continue to forge ahead fearlessly (and if I am honest, sometimes fearfully), embracing each new moment, knowing that I possess the tools to overcome any obstacle that may come my way.

Now, I want to share these three powerful tools with you— tools that helped me find relief and hope. Tools that will empower you to take steps toward breaking free from anxiety and mental health struggles one day and, sometimes, one moment at a time:

1. **STORIES** - Within you lies a profound power—the ability to rewrite your narrative and redefine your reality. When fear and negativity threaten to overwhelm

your mind, listen to a playlist of uplifting audio and motivational talks. These voices will stand as unwavering allies, replacing the limiting beliefs that once held you captive. Embrace this liberating truth: Life is not happening to you; it's happening for you and through you.

2.  **FOCUS** - Gratitude is a magical force that can liberate you from fear. Take a few moments each morning and night to acknowledge even one thing you are grateful for that day. Redirect your thoughts away from what you lack and toward the abundance around you. Embrace the power of positive focus and watch as it transforms your perspective and attracts more blessings into your life.

3.  **CURIOSITY** - Be curious about your emotions and struggles. Seek to understand the workings of your brain and emotions. Reach out for support and guidance, and approach your challenges with compassion and a willingness to learn and grow. Embrace the journey of self-discovery and resilience, knowing it is a transformative path toward healing.

## 1. STORIES

Back then, I felt like a victim of life happening to me—a never-ending barrage of assaults. To counter this, every time I felt scared, overwhelmed, or panicked, I would play one of the audios on a loop. I would immerse myself in the words being said, replacing the doom-filled narrative that relentlessly ran through my mind. Sometimes, even in the middle of the night, I would seek relief through these audios.

Now, many years later, I understand that when we allow negative, self-limiting, or destructive thoughts to dominate our minds, we unintentionally invite those qualities to manifest in our reality. Our thoughts act as a filter, influencing our perceptions, attitudes, and actions. They shape our beliefs about ourselves, others, and the world around us, impacting how we show up in our relationships, careers, and overall well-being.

Inspired by Albert Einstein's insight, "We cannot solve our problems with the same thinking we used when we created them," I recognized the urgent need to change the narrative in my mind. I turned to Tony Robbins' Ultimate Edge program and Esther Hicks' Rampages of Appreciation to do this.

To hear someone else's voice in my head other than my insecure, fearful one, I made it a habit to play an audio whenever I felt frozen in place and panicking. Sometimes, I would listen to them on a loop for hours to find that two millimeters of relief.

Through this powerful tool of *stories*, I slowly reshaped my self-perception and adopted different empowering stories and dialogue. These two-millimeter shifts in mindset opened doors to new possibilities, fueled personal growth, and allowed me to approach panic, overwhelm, and challenges with fresh perspectives.

By rewriting my narrative, I tapped into my true potential and began to solve problems from a place of expanded awareness. The transformative journey of storytelling continues to shape my life. Today, I no longer believe that life is happening to me. I choose to believe it is happening for me and through me.

In his book *As A Man Thinketh*, James Allen said, "He thinks in secret, and it comes to pass: Environment is but his looking glass." This idea aligns with Hermetic Philosophy's principle that "as within, so without, as above, so below, as the universe, so the soul." Both highlight the notion that our external experiences and circumstances are a reflection of our internal thoughts, beliefs, and attitudes. They suggest that our inner world and mindset shape our external reality and the events we attract into our lives.

To change our circumstances, we must change our inner dialogues. Creating a playlist on YouTube can provide a constant source of inspiration and motivation to support this inner transformation. By curating a collection of uplifting audios, we reinforce positive narratives and align ourselves with our desired reality.

Here are some links to some great audios that you can carry around with you and play throughout the day:

- Esther Hicks: My Dominant Intent (https://youtu. be/6hGjP7rqDNc)
- Esther Hicks: Good Morning Rampage (https://youtu. be/FmczMP1gQzk)
- Esther Hicks: Everything is Always Working Out for Me (https://youtu.be/3ae4vdLKon4)
- Charlie Harary: Change the Audio Series (http:// idezzinemylife.org/real-change.html)
- Tony Robbins: Motivation (https://youtu.be/ QZvt4epqY9g)

\* \* \*

## 2. FOCUS

> *"Our brain cannot hold more than one thought at a time. FEAR or LOVE."*
>
> – Marianne Williamson

In those moments of debilitating fear and anxiety, I couldn't see a way out of the labyrinth that felt like it was closing in on me. But I discovered a powerful tool: Focusing on anything other than fear. Our brains are not hardwired to focus simultaneously on specific, day-to-day activities and more collective, long-term objectives.

M.I.T. featured research from Morela Hernandez, associate professor at Darden School of Business, University of Virginia, that demonstrated our brain cannot focus on two things simultaneously.

That means when I feel fear, if I can focus on anything else, my brain cannot keep me in fear. The magic word to get me out of fear? *Gratitude.*

Gratitude holds a miraculous power that can liberate us from the clutches of fear. It's an awe-inspiring revelation rooted in the fascinating realm of neurological science. As wondrous as it is, our brilliant human brain cannot focus on two things at once. It's wired in such a way that when we deliberately cultivate gratitude, fear has no choice but to step aside.

Isn't that remarkable? By consciously choosing to embrace gratitude, we effortlessly shift our mental landscape. We redirect our thoughts away from fear and invite a profound sense of appreciation and positivity into our hearts. It's like flipping a switch, transforming darkness into light.

Something truly magical happens when we immerse ourselves in the warmth of gratitude. We transcend our worries and anxieties. We break free from the limitations that fear imposes upon us. Suddenly, our perspective broadens, and we start seeing the beauty and abundance surrounding us. Gratitude becomes our guiding star, our sanctuary amidst life's storms.

It gently reminds us to focus on the blessings we have rather than being consumed by what we lack. It opens our eyes to the miracles that unfold before us, both big and small.

*"What you focus on expands."*

– Oprah Winfrey

*"What you focus on grows, what you think about expands, and what you dwell upon determines your destiny."*

– Robin Sharma

The concept that what we focus on expands is rooted in the idea that our thoughts and attention have the power to shape our experiences and reality. When we consistently direct our attention and energy toward a particular subject or goal, we tend to notice more related opportunities, insights, and possibilities in our lives.

Psychologically, this phenomenon is supported by the Reticular Activating System (RAS) in our brains. The RAS acts as a filter, determining which information from our surroundings is important and deserving of our attention. By consciously focusing on a specific goal or mindset, we activate the RAS to be more attuned to relevant information, leading us to notice and attract more of what aligns with our focus.

Scientific studies on the brain have shown that focused attention can strengthen neural connections associated with specific tasks or thought patterns. This neuronal plasticity suggests that the more we focus on particular thoughts or actions, the more our brain reinforces and expands those neural pathways, making them more accessible and automatic over time.

Daily focusing on gratitude can remarkably transform our lives from the inside out. It's an invitation to experience the profound shift that occurs when we cultivate an attitude of appreciation.

**Here's a practical way to infuse your days with gratitude**: Take a few moments each morning and at night before drifting off to sleep. Begin by writing down just one thing you're grateful for. It could be as simple as a warm cup of tea or a loving gesture from a friend. As you continue, gradually build up to listing three things, and then ten, that you're grateful for in those precious moments.

You'll be astounded by the profound impact this simple, yet powerful practice will have on your life. You'll discover an abundant wellspring of joy and contentment by consciously focusing on the blessings surrounding you. Your perspective will shift, and even amidst life's challenges, you'll find a deep sense of gratitude for the lessons they bring.

This beautiful gratitude ritual becomes a transformative tool, gradually shaping how you perceive the world. It uplifts your spirits, nurtures a positive mindset, and attracts even more blessings into your life.

So, embrace the power of focusing on gratitude. Dedicate those precious moments each morning and night to acknowledging the blessings that grace your life. Let gratitude be your guiding light, and watch as it illuminates your path, opening doors to a life brimming with joy, abundance, and limitless possibilities.

\* \* \*

## 3. CURIOSITY

*"Curiosity warms up these circuits and the hippocampus to prepare the brain to learn and create long-term memories."*

– Dr. Judy Willis

Let's talk about the amazing impact of curiosity. When I was trapped in a never-ending loop of anxiety and disastrous "What if?" scenarios, fueling my already heightened fear and anxiety,

I discovered the simple but profound power of curiosity. It wasn't about hype or excitement; it was about finding a lifeline.

To cope with my overwhelming emotions, I turned to journaling every day. It became a safe space where I could pour out my thoughts and gently explore their reasons. In those moments of curiosity, something beautiful happened; I felt a sense of warmth and comfort within myself.

Dr. Judy Willis put it best: "Curiosity is like a gentle spark that warms up our brain, especially the part responsible for creating memories." It allowed me to open my mind and heart to new perspectives and to be receptive to learning and growth.

As I embraced curiosity, I found solace in the release of neurotransmitters like dopamine and norepinephrine. These natural chemicals lifted my spirits, and learning became an inspiring journey rather than a burden.

And here's where things really hit home. My struggles with certain emotions weren't just a lack of willpower or strength. Understanding that my emotional experiences had a physiological basis brought me compassion and a desire to know more about myself.

Dr. Joe Dispenza's explanation of addiction, and the powerful connection between our emotions and our brain chemistry, resonated deeply. It wasn't about blame or judgment; it was about understanding the intricate workings of my brain and emotions.

That started my heartfelt journey of discovery and healing. Curiosity was a quiet force that led me to profound realizations and transformations. I started working with coaches and mentors to help me see the patterns I couldn't see. They helped me approach my struggles with compassion and understanding, embracing the delicate balance of emotions and brain chemistry.

Remember, these tools may seem simple, but their impact is profound. I want you to know that your struggles do not define you. You have the power inside of you to make that two-millimeter shift and step into a life of empowerment, joy, and limitless possibilities.

With each stride you take, never forget that you are not alone; the threads of hope and resilience connect us. Within you lies the strength to overcome anxiety and mental health struggles. Embrace these empowering tools, and let them be your compass, guiding you to the relief and liberation you so profoundly deserve. Believe in the boundless power that resides within you, and with that belief, take that brave first step toward transformation. A radiant future awaits you, and I am here, energetically cheering you on as you embark on this transformative journey of self-discovery and healing.

*　　*　　*

An adventurous and resilient soul, Ronita was born in Nigeria, raised in London, and now feels blessed to call Antigua home. Having escaped a toxic marriage, she struggled & embraced single motherhood with her four incredible daughters in Los Angeles, learning profound lessons in love and humility.

Having worked in diverse retail sectors and online platforms, she uncovered her passion for coaching and mentoring. With her innate ability to perceive the unspoken, she assists others in unraveling their stories, gaining profound awareness, and reconnecting them with their inner wisdom.

Once her youngest daughter left for college, she embarked on an island-hopping adventure that eventually brought her to the healing shores of Antigua. Inspired by her transformative experience, she created Master The 8 Experience—a bespoke coaching journey that invites individuals to pause, reflect, and thrive against the enchanting backdrop of the island.

When she's not coaching, you'll find her on the tennis court, immersing herself in languages, exploring cultures, and savoring delectable cuisines. Her vision extends to living and working across 40+ islands, uplifting others, and leaving a trail of happiness and inspiration, echoing the timeless words of Mother Teresa.

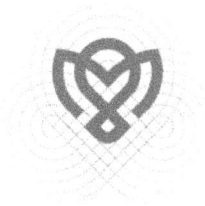

Ronita Godsi
Coach | Educator | Advisor | Mentor
Founder of ReSET and Master The 8
*A bespoke coaching experience on*
*Caribbean island of Antigua*
www.MasterThe8.com

# Love, Meditate, and Celebrate: Don't Let Your Thoughts Overpower You

### By
### Titia Niehorster

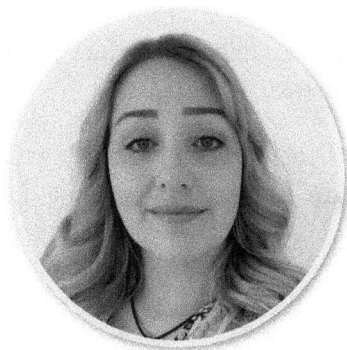

Anxiety can often interfere with our thoughts and emotions throughout our lives, leading us into a state of conflict and fear. However, there is a way to find inner peace and transcendence. This chapter explores the wisdom that has helped me overcome anxiety, inspired by the teachings of several yogis, spiritual masters, and a Course in Miracles.

"Love, Meditate, and Celebrate" are tools that will help you feel more love and overcome your feelings of fear.

"If someone else can do it, you can do it, too," is something I always have told myself when facing a challenge. This affirmation has helped me a lot, from childbirth to starting my business.

Yet there still were moments when I felt lost in anxiety and worries.

In these moments, my thoughts seemed to take over, and I felt anxiety expand throughout my mind and body.

I didn't like feeling this way, and one of my tactics to deal with this was to keep myself busy. I learned how to do this when I became a single mom and had to provide for my young children. Of course, being a mom of six children helped fill my calendar, but it was also the perfect excuse not to face my feelings or take time for myself.

Social media was another distraction. Having a large following gave me certain obligations to post daily and grow my audience.

But there came a point when I couldn't distract myself from dealing with my feelings any longer. I felt overwhelmed and stressed, knowing I had to change something. I felt it in every bone of my body; I needed to heal. And I needed to get out of the rat race to heal. And so began my spiritual journey.

Over the years, I researched and tried several self-help techniques, but I couldn't find one that helped me deal with feelings of anxiety.

It was a combination of several techniques and steps that became the right path for me to transform my feelings of anxiety.

The first step is to understand anxiety. Anxiety arises from different causes: uncertainty, past traumas, fear of the future, or even unresolved conflicts within ourselves. Anxiety primarily occurs when we identify with the ego, which thrives on separation and judgement. To break free from anxiety, we must seek a higher perspective, transcending the ego.

1.   Other people's behavior says something about them—not about me.

I learned this during my mediation education. No matter the situation, we can always choose how we react and behave toward others and ourselves. If someone is rude to you, this says something about them—not you.

This realization lifted a weight off my shoulders because I could get down and anxious when someone misbehaved toward me. Knowing this made me feel more free and much less anxious, giving me more confidence to communicate with and approach people.

2.   "We are where our thoughts are."

My second step in overcoming anxiety was learning that we are not our thoughts.

This realization meant true liberation for me. As I mentioned before, I have had moments where I could feel overpowered by fear-based thoughts.

Knowing that we are not our thoughts means we can influence our minds.

Therefore, becoming overpowered by fear-based thoughts is not needed at all.

We can change and control this.

In my search for self-development, I learned that we are where our thoughts are.

Say this aloud several times: "We are where our thoughts are."

Truly realize this. This means that when we're thinking fear-based thoughts, there is a good chance we will start feeling anxious.

3. Think with intention.

To change, we need to start by witnessing our thoughts without judgement. This is known as mindfulness in the West, and in the East, witness consciousness. Become a witness to your thoughts, an observer, if you will.

If you conclude that you don't like your thoughts, you can then decide to change them.

Start to think with intention. No longer let thinking passively happen to you. Instead, take charge and choose to think the thoughts you want.

4. Choose the right mind.

The mind of conflict and fear tempts us with limiting beliefs and negative self-talk. It often seeks to sabotage our progress toward inner peace and spiritual growth. To choose the right mind is to align ourselves with the divine source of love, wisdom, and healing. It requires a conscious effort to reject fear-based thoughts and not be passively drawn into the wrong mind of conflict and fear.

Choose your right mind of love, compassion, and forgiveness, and embrace the truth of our innate worthiness and connection.

By becoming aware of your thoughts and observing them, you know whether they serve you. If they are not serving you, choose the thoughts that do serve you.

5.   In the present moment, we can find peace.

Mindfulness or witness consciousness plays a crucial role in overcoming anxiety. By observing our thoughts without judgment, we can identify anxiety triggers and gradually release their hold on us.

I need to emphasize the importance of staying present while practicing this. In the present moment, we can find peace and release ourselves from the burdens of the past or the worries about the future.

6.   When life gives you lemons, take the zest and turn them into positive learning moments.

We all know that life is not without its challenges; it presents us with lemons—difficulties and setbacks. Even though they can be bitter to taste, just like lemons, these challenges carry a zest that enhances flavors. Extract the essence of positivity and growth from life's adversities.

I have learned, and I encourage you to view these challenging moments as opportunities for learning and transformation. Become an optimist; choose the positive in different situations. Replace negative thoughts with positive ones. The glass is half empty, but it's also half full.

By repeating this, positivity becomes second nature.

Making this a habit will create new neuro-pathways in your brain, creating new habits and behaviors.

Remember: You are where your thoughts are. So it is best to focus on the positive.

    7.  Choose love. Fear is always a lie.

Our Truth is Love.

If you have fear-based thoughts, know these are not your truth. Fear is always a lie; it is merely an illusion.

Some say FEAR means: False Expectations Appearing Real, which fits the description.

The opposite of fear—the antidote—is love. You can transform your fear-based thoughts to love and find your truth there.

In truth, all is well, and there is no need to be afraid of anything. In truth, you are perfect just the way you are, and you don't need to change anything about yourself.

You are fully loved and accepted as you are.

Love is the essence that connects us all. We can resolve anything with love. When we start sowing more love within ourselves and extend this to others, we break down the walls of separation that grow anxiety and conflict. Love becomes our guiding emotion, leading us towards more unity and compassion, empowering us to embrace life with open hearts.

    8.  Rome wasn't built in a day, and the same goes for creating new habits of thinking.

When you apply these techniques and release yourself from fear-based thoughts, there might come a day when you suddenly feel anxiety again. If that happens, don't worry about it; more importantly, don't give up. It is a process to adjust to this new way of intentional thinking. Be patient with yourself.

Rome wasn't built in a day, and the same goes for creating new habits of thinking. Most importantly, don't judge yourself for feeling this way; instead, forgive yourself. Love and forgiveness of the self are crucial steps in overcoming anxiety.

Forgive yourself and realize that these are just thoughts, and these thoughts are lies.

These are not your truth. These thoughts and feelings are not who you are and will not become your reality.

Start again by observing them and deciding they are not what you choose. Keep replacing your fear-based thoughts and emotions with love and the positive thoughts of your choice.

Choose consciously who you are, who you want to be, and what thoughts are helping you. Write them down if you wish to, and repeat them several times daily.

Take some time to become quiet every day and spend time reading the thoughts you want to think and how you want to feel.

9. Practice gratitude.

Do you want to feel more happiness? Ask yourself: *How does a happy person feel?*

Happy people are often grateful and think about everything they can be grateful for.

By being grateful for even the smallest blessings and focusing on gratitude, we open ourselves to a deeper appreciation of life, giving us opportunities to uncover hidden blessings.

Repeating positive affirmations, such as "I am love," "I am safe," and "I am worthy," can gradually rewire our thought patterns, leading us away from anxiety and towards self-empowerment.

There are many things to be grateful for, such as:

I am grateful to have a roof over my head.

- I am grateful to have food on the table every day.
- I am grateful to have clean water to drink every day.
- I am grateful to be in good health.
- I love life, and life loves me.

Start writing some affirmations that help you.

Remember that your words are important; they carry energy and can add positive energy to your life, so choose them with care and love.

10. Meditate.

When I first learned about meditation, I thought this would take me several hours a day. Because I thought meditation would take me several hours a day to do right, I hesitated to practice for a long time.

Taking some time for yourself to become quiet every day to practice choosing the thoughts you want to think and how you want to feel can be a challenge for busy people.

Some people meditate one to two hours every day. However, there are many ways to take some quiet time, and there is more than one way to meditate. If sitting quietly for one to two hours a day isn't for you, don't worry. It's not for me, either.

Meditation is a great tool to find inner stillness in the chaos of our minds and busy lives. By sitting in silence, observing our thoughts without judgement, we create space for peace and clarity to emerge. In the stillness of meditation, we connect with our true selves, the witness of our thoughts, and realize that we are not at the mercy of our anxious minds.

Taking quiet time can be as easy as taking a short walk in nature, enjoying the view from your balcony, listening to the birds sing, lying down for a moment, listening to calming music, or using the time before you fall asleep or wake up. Whatever appeals to you.

The point is to dedicate some time when it's convenient for you and your lifestyle.

Expanding your quiet time can be a process. When you notice an improvement in your thinking, you'll be eager to progress even more. Start small and work your way up.

Don't worry about it if you don't have time some days. Have fun, laugh at yourself, and don't take it all too seriously.

You're human, and you're not meant to be flawless.

We try. We watch. We learn. We take a step back. We move forward, practice, and build progress along the way.

11. Celebrate.

Living in the past or constantly worrying about the future only strengthens anxiety. Celebration is a practice of honoring the present moment and embracing life with joy and gratitude. Instead of allowing anxiety to overshadow our life, we can celebrate its beauty and wonder.

Embrace the present moment and recognize it as the point of power where we can make conscious choices and shape our reality with love. Celebration instills a sense of appreciation.

When you adopt an attitude of gratitude, you'll have so much to celebrate. Take the time to celebrate the little moments and successes. For example, celebrate being one week fear free after applying some of the techniques from this book. Teach them to your kids and celebrate their success. Go out and have yourself a fancy coffee with a friend, bake cookies with your kids, treat yourself with flowers, or cook your partner's favorite meal.

Fill your life with happy memories of little moments.

12. Shift your perception; overcome the illusion of separation.

While you're living your life and overcoming these feelings and thoughts of fear, there might be moments when you believe you're the only one feeling this way. It's easy to think that you're the only one feeling this way or that the world is scary and unsafe.

I know I felt this way many times. However, this was an error of judgement on my part.

Since then, I have learned an important cause of anxiety is the belief in separation from others, the world, and the divine. The illusion of separation creates fear, as we feel alone, disconnected, and vulnerable. However, the truth is that we are all connected, and the source of love is within us all. Recognizing this truth will show you that anxiety is an illusion because fear cannot flourish in oneness.

To change this view of the world being a hostile and threatening place, we can choose to view our world through the lens of compassion and unity. Recognizing that we are where our thoughts are, and our perception shapes our reality, we can intentionally replace fear-based thoughts with thoughts of love.

When you look at the world and all the people sharing it with you, it's important to remember that we are all equal and here to live our lives to the best of our knowledge, wishes, and desires. We are not all at the same place in life.

Living in a country where it's hard to survive is very different from living in a country where clean water and housing are available to everyone. Being born into a loving family is very different from being born into an area with war and conflict. This is crucial to remember when you see and encounter other people.

Look at others from a place of love and compassion—not pity—and without judgement. We can never know how someone feels, what they have experienced, and why they do the things they do. What motivates them is only something they know. And maybe they're not even conscious of that.

When we're not in a state of witness consciousness, we do so many things on autopilot—subconsciously.

We all live our lives according to what we experience and learn along the way.

From our parents, friends, families, schools, religions, political systems, cultures, and countries. This means we're all operating from our unique perspectives.

13. The power of forgiveness

Look at everyone as someone who needs love, and forgive them when they're not behaving according to how you want them to.

Looking at people this way, you will find that you're much less likely to engage in conflict.

This is easy to practice when people are nice to you. It's not easy when someone is rude to you and wants to draw you into conflict, gossiping, or other types of negativity.

When this happens, remember that conflict and negativity are not your choices, and intentionally choose the mind of peace.

It helps to pause before you react. This way, you can choose to respond from the mind of peace rather than reacting from the mind of conflict.

The power of forgiveness does not mean condoning or excusing harmful actions but rather releasing ourselves from the burden of carrying resentment and anger. By forgiving others and ourselves, we unravel the thoughts of anxiety, allowing space for healing and transformation.

Remember, life is a beautiful journey filled with ups and downs, and when it gives us lemons, we have the power to turn them into positive learning moments. By practicing witness consciousness, we can start to think intentionally and transform our fear-based thoughts into thoughts of love, remembering that our truth is love, and fear is always a lie.

By sowing more love and compassion into our hearts and adopting a forgiving nature toward ourselves and others, we break down the illusions of separation that grow anxiety and conflict. Love becomes our guiding emotion, leading us towards more unity and compassion, empowering us to embrace life with open hearts.

By consciously building quiet time for ourselves in our days, step by step, we can learn to choose our right mind of peace in many encounters with ourselves and others.

Spending more time celebrating our successes will fill our lives with more joy. This way, we can guide ourselves toward the path of a beautiful, anxiety-free life filled with inner peace, love, unity, and happiness.

Let us all: Love, Meditate, and Celebrate.

# Navigating Stress and Anxiety in Modern Life: How to Find Calm in the Chaos

## By
## Shmiko Cole

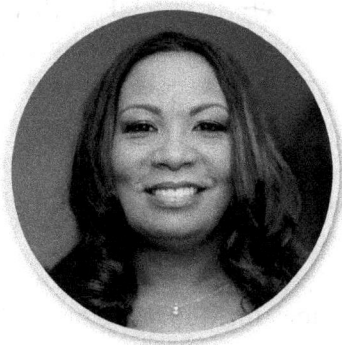

I have worked in corporate America and retail management for nearly three decades and in the competitive workforce in more recent years. I have two adult sons, whom I raised in a city known for its attention to growth, status, and prestige. I was very successful in all facets of my work and business. This success, however, came with a cost: My health and wellness suffered tremendously. I wish I had known then what I know now about how to manage stress levels positively. Fast forward to today, and you'll see a different person. As a now-seasoned veteran of balancing personal and business life, I am happily in control of my well-being more than ever before. I wish to pass on what I know to whom it will support and serve best: young, eager businesspeople wishing to succeed in both work and family life.

The high-level business workplace is known for its intense competition, demanding responsibilities, and high expectations. As individuals climb the corporate ladder or take on significant leadership roles in business, the pressures and stressors they face increase exponentially. Stress at this high level is a pervasive issue that affects the physical and mental well-being of employees, leaders, and business owners. This stress greatly hampers organizational productivity and performance. In today's corporate climate, understanding how to navigate stress effectively is crucial to thriving and growing your business and developing a healthy personal life. Many people speak about the adverse outcomes that prolonged stress can cause, but I prefer to look at the positive side. I choose to focus on achievable positive results instead. When stress is managed effectively, it can lead to numerous physical and mental benefits.

I.   Positive Outcomes of Managing Stress Effectively

- Improved Mental Health: Chronic stress can negatively impact mental health, leading to anxiety, depression, and other mood disorders. By managing stress, individuals will experience improved emotional well-being and greater resilience when facing life's challenges.

- Enhanced Physical Health: Stress can harm the body. Elevated blood pressure, weakened immune function, and increased risk of heart disease all result from unmanaged tension. Managing stress can help lower these risks and promote overall physical health.

- Better Sleep: High stress levels often result in difficulty falling or staying asleep. Stress management techniques can improve sleep quality, helping individuals feel more rested and rejuvenated.

- Increased Productivity: When stress becomes overwhelming, it can hinder concentration, focus, and productivity. Managing stress can help individuals regain their ability to concentrate and work more efficiently.

- Enhanced Decision-Making: Stress can cloud judgment and lead to impulsive decisions. By managing stress, individuals can think more clearly and make better decisions, both in personal and professional settings.

- Strengthened Relationships: High stress levels can lead to irritability and conflict. Managing stress can improve communication and foster healthier connections with others.

- Reduced Risk of Burnout: Chronic stress contributes to burnout, affecting various aspects of life, including work, relationships, and personal well-being. Managing stress helps prevent burnout and fosters a better work-life balance.

- Lowered Risk of Mental Health Disorders: Effective stress management can reduce the risk of developing or exacerbating mental health conditions, protecting the mind.

- Improved Coping Skills: Individuals develop effective coping skills by learning how to manage stress effectively, enabling them to handle future challenges with greater ease and resilience.

- Better Overall Quality of Life: Ultimately, managing stress leads to improved well-being, greater satisfaction with life, and a more positive outlook on the future.

## II. Chief Causes of Stress in the High-Level Workplace

- Workload and Responsibilities: High-level professionals often shoulder immense workloads and responsibilities. Long working hours, tight deadlines, and a constant need to deliver top-quality results create significant pressure that can be overwhelming.

- High Expectations: Executives and leaders must lead by example and consistently meet or exceed targets. The fear of failure and the desire to maintain a flawless image can intensify stress levels.

- Decision-Making Pressure: High-level professionals continually face critical decision-making situations that impact the company's future. The weight of these decisions can lead to anxiety and stress.

- Uncertainty and Change: Constant change and uncertainty characterize the corporate business environment. Leaders must adapt quickly to new challenges, which can lead to chronic stress.

- Interpersonal Challenges: Managing teams and interacting with diverse personalities can be challenging. Handling conflicts and maintaining effective communication adds to the stress experienced by high-level professionals.

## III. Effects of Stress in the High-Level Workplace

- Health Implications: Stress in the high-level workplace can manifest in physical symptoms like headaches, gastrointestinal issues, and sleep disruption. Prolonged exposure to stress can contribute to serious health problems, including cardiovascular diseases, weakened immune systems, and mental health disorders.

- Reduced Job Satisfaction: While high-level positions often come with prestige and financial rewards, persistent stress can erode job satisfaction. The constant pressure and lack of work-life balance can lead to burnout, diminishing the overall joy of work.

- Decline in Productivity: Stressed employees are more likely to experience reduced focus, creativity, and problem-solving abilities. This decline in productivity can have a cascading effect on the organization's overall performance.

- Employee / Leadership Turnover: Stressful workplaces can result in high employee turnover rates, as professionals may seek opportunities in less demanding environments to improve their well-being.

- Organizational Reputation: A high-stress work culture can negatively impact the organization's reputation and ability to attract and retain top talent. News of a stressful work environment can deter potential applicants and customers or clients.

## IV. Corresponding Coping Strategies for High-Level Workplace Stress

- Implementing Supportive Policies: Organizations should adopt policies that promote work-life balance, flexible working hours, and adequate leave entitlements. Supporting employees' personal lives can alleviate stress and improve overall job satisfaction.

- Encouraging Open Communication: Creating an atmosphere of open communication allows employees to express their concerns and seek assistance when needed. Regular feedback sessions and one-on-one meetings with supervisors can foster trust and provide opportunities to address stressors.

- Providing Stress Management Workshops: Stress management workshops and training programs can equip high-level professionals with practical coping techniques, including mindfulness and time management strategies.

- Building a Supportive Work Culture: Organizational leaders should model healthy behavior and promote a positive work culture emphasizing well-being and mental health. Encouraging teamwork, recognition, and celebrating achievements can contribute to a supportive environment.

- Employee Assistance Programs (EAPs): Implementing EAPs can offer employees confidential support and counseling services, allowing them to address stress-related concerns and seek professional help.

Stress in the high-level workplace is a significant issue that harms individuals and organizations. The demanding nature of these roles, coupled with high expectations and constant pressure, can lead to adverse health effects, decreased productivity, and organizational challenges. By implementing supportive policies, promoting open communication, and offering stress management resources, organizations can help their professionals better cope with pressure, fostering a healthier and more productive work environment. Addressing stress in the high-level workplace is not only essential for the well-being of employees but also for the long-term success of the organization.

Everything you just read is about how organizations can reduce collective stress. But what about you, the individual? What can you do to ensure that you aren't spreading yourself too thin and are caring for your physical and mental health in the long term?

As you know, you can't pour from an empty cup. Sometimes, I think that adage does us a disservice as it makes us feel that we can fill another's cup with just a few drops on our own. Technically, yes, you can, but what good is that serving to you or anyone else? Ideally, we should all keep our proverbial cups as full as possible. I know this may sound unrealistic with some of the workloads you face, but I encourage you to *make time to address your stress load.* In some form or another, our actions have consequences, which goes for lack of effort, too. Just as you can't keep your car running efficiently without regular maintenance and frequent refueling, you can't keep putting off the needs of your body and mind. I've chosen seven tips that have helped me most along my journey, full of trial and error.

V.  Personal Stress Coping Strategies

- Set Realistic Goals: Break down large tasks into smaller, manageable steps. Setting achievable goals will prevent you from becoming overwhelmed and keep you moving forward. Remember that setting realistic goals doesn't mean settling for mediocrity. It's about balancing challenging yourself and being practical about what you can accomplish. Setting realistic goals increases your chances of success and builds confidence in your ability to achieve your goals.

- Limit Technology Use: Set boundaries on your screen time and create designated periods for digital detox. Constant exposure to social media and news can contribute to stress, so giving yourself breaks is essential.

- Challenge Negative Thoughts: Identify negative thought patterns and challenge their accuracy. Replace them with more positive and constructive perspectives.

You can develop a more balanced and realistic view by questioning and challenging negative thoughts. Remember that challenging negative thoughts takes practice and persistence. It's a skill you can hone over time. The more you work on it, the more you train new neural pathways geared toward positive thinking.

- Learn to Say No: This one can be hard in business, but it is so important. Recognize your limits, and don't overcommit yourself. Saying no to additional responsibilities or social engagements when you're already feeling overwhelmed is okay. Saying no allows you to be more intentional with your choices. It helps you make decisions based on what aligns with your values and long-term objectives. Saying no respectfully and assertively fosters better communication with others. It shows that you value honesty and openness in your relationships. Learning how to get better and better at it is a practice. Before long, you will remember that you have control over your choices and are not obligated to please everyone.

- Practice Mindfulness: Be present in the moment and cultivate awareness of your thoughts and emotions. Mindfulness techniques, such as meditation and deep breathing exercises, can help you stay grounded during stressful situations. Besides stress reduction, mindfulness techniques can manage and alleviate pain, boost the immune system, develop greater resilience, lower blood pressure, improve sleep quality, and boost creativity. These days, you can find all kinds of apps or go to YouTube University and easily find mindfulness practices that suit your lifestyle and belief systems.

- Engage in Physical Activity: I'm not asking you to train for a marathon or join a fitness club. The trick is to do something you enjoy, at least a little. Regular exercise, whether going to the gym, hiking, practicing yoga, or dancing, releases endorphins and reduces stress. Find an activity you enjoy and make it a part of your routine. Outside activities are especially effective and rewarding.

- Seek Social Support: Share your feelings with trusted friends, family members, subject experts, or a therapist. Talking about your stress and anxiety can help you gain perspective and receive support. It can also release tension by sharing and getting it all out. Expressing your emotions can provide relief and bring a fresh take on your situation.

- Practice Gratitude: The benefits of the practice of gratitude are quantifiable. Grateful individuals tend to have a more optimistic view of life, improving overall psychological well-being. Incorporating gratitude into one's life can be done in various ways, such as keeping a gratitude journal, verbally expressing thanks to others, reflecting on positive experiences, or even taking a moment each day to acknowledge and appreciate the good things in life. Take a few minutes each day to reflect on what you are grateful for. Gratitude exercises can shift your focus from negative thoughts to positive aspects of life.

Remember that managing stress, anxiety, and mental health is a personal life-long journey, and seeking professional help is encouraged if you find it challenging to move forward on your own. Be patient with yourself and celebrate your progress, small and large. Step by step, intentionally implement new healthy habits, and you'll be on your way to finding more well-being and balance. Again, seek ideas, access, and resources from the experts in your field. These are some of the most fruitful practices that have worked for me.

Start immediately and do something that will create an impact. I speak often about the balance, even in business between the head and the heart. All decisions that you make should consider both how the critical wise brain thinks about it, and also how your heart thinks about it. We may operate often in technical and fast paced business environments, yet in the end, we are all human, and our humanity has its own lenses for decision making. The world will continue to give us potential stressors, and we must consistently discover ways to neutralize and eliminate them.

I wish you much success on your path to empowerment and positive work-life integration. Stay amazing, beautiful people!

# DEALING WITH WHAT IS, NOT WHAT WAS

BY
TIM BOWMAN

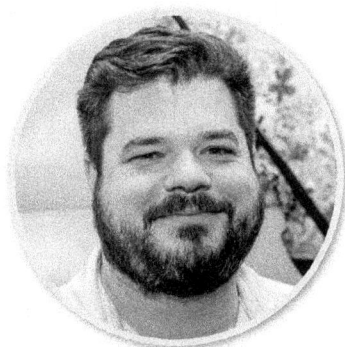

Thank you for taking the time to read this book and my chapter contributing to it. Your time is valuable, and I appreciate your willingness to spend some of it hearing what I have to say. I'm not a therapist, and I don't even pretend to have everything together in a nice, neat box. What I do have is some perspective on how my past has informed my tendencies to act or react in stressful situations; how my personal experiences, generational traumas of my family, and economic status when I was young have built patterns of behavior on which I have relied until very recently; and just how much all of that doesn't serve me in my present or in pursuing my desired future.

You may have heard of the term Xennial, which describes a microgeneration of people born between 1977 and 1983 in Western societies. I fall directly in the middle of this time frame and certainly share the traits that describe us as having an analog childhood and digital youth. We experienced the bootstraps mentality of the 80s, being left to our own devices for most of the day while our parents tried to scratch out a living. It was important not to be a burden or even really noticed too much, and self-sufficiency was expected as early as possible.

My family, which was blended and broken multiple times in my youth, experienced hardship in the form of needing government assistance at times, often moving to try to better our position, and building family businesses to ultimately achieve some financial stability. All these things combined to create someone who desperately tries not to rock the boat while only trying to be seen as being useful, exceptional, or exemplary.

My parents did the best they could with the upbringing and circumstances of their lives, but there are traumas and learned behaviors on their part that run deep. I don't blame them for acting on their upbringings, but it naturally affected how I perceived the world and built my responses—consciously and subconsciously—to it.

I grew up the youngest of four, all of whom have powerful personalities. You've read a chapter in this book from one of them. We all experienced our traumas and challenges, of which others may or may not have been aware. One way I tried to keep my life as easy as possible was to recognize what was getting my older siblings in trouble and avoid those activities.

I started working for my mom's small business at six, going to the shop after school multiple days a week to craft items, sort inventory, prepare for sales or trips, and be useful in any other way I could. I would travel with her and my stepdad to auctions on weekends during the school year and in the summers to various fairs, setting up the booth and helping with sales. These things brought me a lot of fun experiences, including meeting and helping other vendors when times were slow, for which I remain grateful. However, they were a lot of work and not easy. This is one of the things that reinforced the hustle mentality, which is typical of Millennials.

I am not giving all the details of my life here. I only have so much space in this chapter, and there are things you don't need to understand where I'm coming from. Many readers will recognize the influence of the outside world I'm describing here. Hopefully, you have at least found some touch points that will allow you to empathize with a person who grew up pushing down personal desires to maintain peace, who believed that others' desires were more important than his needs, and who did not know what he truly wanted, let alone how to achieve it.

Like most people in the time of sheltering in place and COVID precautions, my life changed dramatically in 2020. The world shutdown and precautions complicated daily activities, and my partner and I had already made plans to move from Los Angeles to Salt Lake City. I was figuring out how to be a remote employee in a hard-hit industry for a supervisor who wasn't the most comfortable with adapting to new methods and technologies—at least when it came to employee expectations. It was stressful and challenged me on personal and professional levels.

At the turn from 2021 into 2022, I was extremely anxious, depressed, and unsure how to move forward after a stressful homebuying experience, multiple deaths in the family, and helping a performing arts organization get back on stage for a live audience after almost two years. I nearly had a breakdown; I wasn't functioning anywhere close to my normal capacity. Finally, I sought long-term therapy and was open to medication to help me with issues that had existed from my earliest memories.

Change wasn't, and still isn't, easy. There isn't a quick fix to anything. If you've made it this far in this book, you probably realize that already. Each day is a challenge—a new struggle but also a new opportunity. This is the great "revelation" I have had this past year and more since I started working heavily on my mental health. I put revelation in quotes because it's advice I have given others for so long. Perhaps, like me, you find yourself much better at giving good advice than taking it—even the advice you would give yourself if you were anyone else. So, with the preamble over, the empathetic part of this chapter, let's talk about some things I want you to understand.

No matter what you have thought of yourself in the past, what others—or yourself—have convinced you to believe, today, you can choose something different. You can actively be the voice in your head and silence the old one. The circumstances, traumas, coping mechanisms, and conditioned responses that have controlled your life only have power if you continue to let them. And you don't have to be perfect at changing the narrative simultaneously.

My six-year-long relationship ended in October of last year. We had a home together, two wonderful dogs, friendships, and family relationships we had built together; very suddenly, that was all gone. My life was falling around me, so I fell into old patterns of getting through the days. I shut strong emotions down, continued in patterns of behavior that didn't acknowledge my needs, and maintained as pleasant an outward appearance as possible. It was exhausting. By the time we re-homed our dogs in early February, I was running on emotional fumes. My work life was suffering. My attendance was unreliable; my focus (what little a person with ADHD has most days) was gone, and I felt terrible about my contributions. Luckily, I now have a boss who has been through many rough patches and understands where I was coming from enough to give me the grace to figure things out.

I realized that part of the attendance issues was due to my medications working. In the past, I had relied on my untreated anxiety to spur me out of bed in the morning or panicked, last-minute excellence to drive me when a deadline was approaching. Now that it was being effectively medicated, which was a relief in almost every way, I had to develop healthy habits to help myself feel motivated. My therapist and I came up with simple things I could do to help get myself to bed at a reasonable time and get me out of bed in the morning, to set reminders for those things that will never actually become habits for me, to leverage the "hit of dopamine" (my therapist's words) I receive by checking things off a list. There are still some days when the old "I shouldn't have to trick myself" voice comes around, but I can usually tell him to shut up. This is what I need *now*, and this is what works *now*, so there isn't any such thing as "should" here.

During this period after the breakup, I finally allowed myself to be diagnosed with ADHD. You probably think that's a funny way to phrase it, but I had known all the symptoms that fit the diagnosis for decades. I'm neither unintelligent nor inobservant, so, of course, I knew, but I grew up in a time where diagnosis and treatment of mental health issues were admissions of weakness. That was the story I heard and internalized.

Finally, freeing myself of that lie, I could seek treatment. The first medication we tried for ADHD didn't help; I even had some deleterious side effects. It was tempting to chuck in the towel and tell myself to just leave it, but I decided not to. I wanted to give myself the best chance to get *better,* not just stop being worse. So, my prescriber and I started another treatment. This one is working. I wouldn't go so far as to say I feel normal—whatever that is—but I feel like I can control my focus most days; hyperfocus is rare, and the frenetic energy is much more limited. The fears I had about feeling suppressed by drugs have not manifested. This is not to say I don't still have days when the old voice taunts me for needing medication; I absolutely do. But now I can recognize that voice as false. This is what I need *now,* so it is what I am doing now.

As I have started quieting the voices and conditioning of the past, my future has started asking for more attention. Much of my life has been spent dealing with one crisis or trauma after another—some of my creation, some circumstances of conditioned responses, some just random life happenings. Through all of it, I can't really complain because it got me to where I am now. Even if that feels like, at 43, I'm just starting my life earnestly. For the first time, I realistically look to the future with an eye for manifesting what I want instead of ridding myself of what I don't want.

Read that again. Ask yourself that question: "How much of my plans for the future are built around achieving what I want rather than getting rid of what I don't want?" It's a powerful, if subtle, question.

Many people, including me until recently, don't even know it's a question they must ask. We are so wrapped up in daily living that it seems ludicrous to ask what we want. The bills must be paid, family cared for, chores done, and various other social obligations met; who has time to think about what they want? You need to make that time. There are tools to help; many of them are described in other chapters of this book. Whether you find your calm in meditation, exercise, spiritual pursuits, or some other activity, it is imperative you find that calm. Only in that calm can you truly examine what has been motivating you. Without that introspection, you cannot move forward proactively.

Take the time to recognize the things that you are doing that are completely products of your past. You don't have to please your parents anymore, fear your teachers, or camouflage yourself from the bullies at school. I guarantee there are daily behaviors you have put in place that directly result from these things. Your parents no longer have any power over your life other than what you give them. Your teachers have done their job—poorly or well; they have nothing left to teach you. Your bullies have their journeys of discovery to make and don't get to define your life anymore. If there are bullies in your life now—spouses, coworkers, family members, friends, or some other social group—you have the power to give yourself permission to end that association.

Only you have that power. You must take it. And you can do it right now. You don't have to feel bad about not having done it sooner. And you don't have to worry about whether you will do it tomorrow if you don't today. Now is the only thing you have control over, and it's the only thing that has to concern you.

Find out who you are now. Do it with purpose. Do it with compassion for yourself. Do it every day.

Thank you for reading this book. On behalf of the other authors and me, I genuinely appreciate your time. As I said at the beginning of this chapter, your time is valuable. I hope it's a little more valuable to you after having read this.

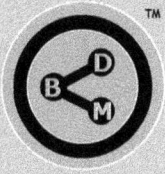

# Bowman Digital Media
## Ira Bowman
### SEO Specialist

951-902-9550

ira@bowmandigitalmedia.com

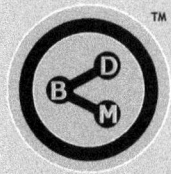

---

## What We Do:

increase sales by generating more website traffic

---

## How We Help:

### SEO:
Search Engine Optimization includes content creation, backlink building, meta data, keyword and traffic monitoring

### Website Development and Maintenance:
We are WordPress Developers

### Graphic Design:
For Print or Online - Logos, Business Cards, Brochures, Custom Design Work

### Photography:
Headshots, Event, Product and Lifestyle

### Videography:
Video Shooting Editing

### Social Media Marketing:
All Platforms Including: LinedIn, Facebook, Instagram, YouTube, Pinterest, Twitter and More.

## Sales Growth by Design

**www.bowmandigitalmedia.com**

www.ingramcontent.com/pod-product-compliance
Lightning Source LLC
Chambersburg PA
CBHW050350280326
41933CB00010BA/1411